Anatomy, Pathophysiology, and Disease Processes - Block 1

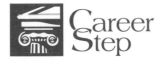

Career Step, LLC
Phone: 801.489.9393
Toll-Free: 800.246.7837
Fax: 801.491.6645
careerstep.com

This text companion contains a snapshot of the online program content converted to a printed format. Please note that the online training program is constantly changing and improving and is always the source of the most up-to-date information.

Product Number: HG-PR-11-003
Generation Date: February 2, 2012

Table of Contents

Unit 1
Introduction

Introduction to Anatomy and Disease, Block 1

Learning Objective

In the first block of *Anatomy and Disease*, the student will learn basic anatomical structures, specifically studying the skeletal, muscular, digestive, respiratory, and reproductive systems. Disease entities, diagnosis, and treatment will also be emphasized as the student is introduced to pathophysiology and disease processes. Throughout this module, illustrations of the various systems and structures will be included to increase student understanding.

Medicine is about people—the minds and bodies of human beings. In the best-case scenario everything works perfectly like a well-oiled machine. In reality, the human body and mind break down and suffer illness and injury. The ravages of the environment, aging, effects of childbirth, overuse, and emotional and physical trauma also affect the human body and mind.

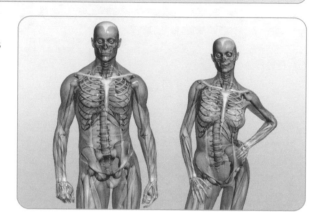

Because medical records document the impact of disease and traumatic events on the body, human anatomy (structure), physiology (function), and disease processes are an important part of medical terminology. A good understanding of the body, its systems, and pathology will prove tremendously helpful to you as a medical worker.

A career in the medical field deals largely with practical application of medical terms. In this setting, a basic understanding of bones, muscles, arteries and veins, ligaments, joints, and organs, as well as body functions (or physiology), such as the respiratory, digestive, and reproductive systems, becomes important. The more terms you are familiar with, the less time you will spend wandering aimlessly through your reference books.

A basic understanding of the anatomy and physiology of the human body, along with the common traumas and diseases that impact it, is essential to understanding key parts of the medical world.

The key word here is basic. Do not be overwhelmed by everything in this module. You are not expected to be a doctor or to know everything that a doctor knows. It is the case, however, that you may be able to easily locate a word in a report because you know the meaning of a word or the location in the body to which a specific term refers.

Unit 2
Anatomy and Disease Basics

Anatomy and Disease Basics – Introduction

This module contains several figures representing different parts and systems of the human body, labeled appropriately, as well as textual information regarding them. Every structure on the figures that is labeled with a number is a term you should be familiar with.

In the following units, you will learn what types of injuries and diseases relate to a particular part of the human body or system. Although there are far too many individual diseases, syndromes, injuries, signs, and treatments for you to learn every one of them, you'll find the most common ones.

Okay—some quick medical humor and then let's get serious about anatomy, physiology, and disease processes.

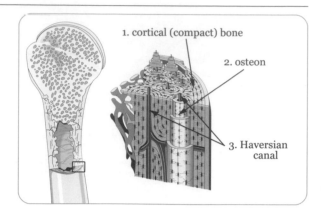

1. cortical (compact) bone
2. osteon
3. Haversian canal

An example of a labeled figure.

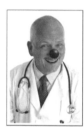

Medical Humor

Doctors were told to contribute to the construction of a new wing at the hospital. What did they do?

The allergists voted to scratch it.
The dermatologists preferred no rash moves.
The gastroenterologists had a gut feeling about it.
The neurologists thought the administration had a lot of nerve.
The obstetricians stated they were laboring under a misconception.
The ophthalmologists considered the idea short-sighted.
The orthopedists issued a joint resolution.
The pathologists yelled, "Over my dead body!"
The pediatricians said, "Grow up."
The proctologists said, "We are in arrears."
The psychiatrists thought it was madness.
The surgeons decided to wash their hands of the whole thing.
The radiologists could see right through it.
The internists thought it was a hard pill to swallow.
The plastic surgeons said, "This puts a whole new face on the matter."
The podiatrists thought it was a big step forward.
The urologists felt the scheme wouldn't hold water.
The cardiologists didn't have the heart to say no.

Levels of Organization

Anatomy refers to the study of the structure of the body. The human body is made up of six levels of structural organization. Each of these levels is related to each other.

The Six Levels of Structural Organization

Chemical **Cellular** **Tissue** **Organ** **System** **Organism**

Level	Structure Definition
Chemical	Atoms and molecules. Atoms such as nitrogen, oxygen, and calcium are essential to the maintenance of life. These atoms combine to form molecules in the body. Examples of molecules are proteins, carbohydrates, fats, and vitamins.
Cellular	Molecules combine to form cells. The cells of the body are the basic structural and functional units of an organism. Examples of cells in the body include muscle cells, nerve cells, and blood cells.
Tissue	Tissues are made up of groups of cells and the materials surrounding them. They work together to perform specific functions. There are four types of tissues in your body. The four types of tissue are: • **epithelial** – Protective tissue found in the linings of cavities and organs and as part of the integumentary system, or skin. This tissue helps to protect the structures it lines from injury and fluid loss. • **muscle** – Responsible for all of the movement of the body. It is subdivided into divisions of skeletal muscle, smooth muscle, and cardiac muscle. Skeletal muscle is made of long fibers and is the tissue that allows for voluntary body movements. Smooth muscle lines the internal organs and carries out primarily involuntary body movements that assist in organ function. Cardiac muscle is found only in the heart and is specifically designed to maintain heartbeat and blood flow • **connective** – Tissue that binds the body together and supports posture and function. This tissue is divided into three subtypes depending on function. Supporting connective tissue consists of the bones and cartilage of the body, which give the body support and base structure. Binding connective tissue is defined as the tendons and ligaments—thick strong tissue that binds muscle to bone and bones to each other. Fibrous connective tissue is also a binding material, though instead of connecting other connective tissues, this tissue connects muscles together and binds the skin to the rest of the body. Adipose, or fat cells, are part of this subdivision serving as a cushioning layer to protect the body. • **nervous** – Composed of nerve cells. It is used as the communication system of the body by passing electronic messages to and from the brain. This allows for all motor functions, both voluntary and involuntary.
Organ	The different kinds of tissue discussed above combine to form the organ level. The organs are composed of two or more types of these tissues. Each organ has specific functions and recognizable shapes. Some examples of organs are the heart, lungs, brain, liver, and kidneys.

System	A system is made up of several organs that have a common function. For example, the organs that are a part of the digestive system break down and absorb food. These organs include the mouth, pharynx (throat), esophagus, stomach, small intestine, and large intestine. Some organs can be part of more than one system. For example, the pancreas is part of both the digestive system and the endocrine system.
Organism	The largest structural level is the organism level. All the parts which make up the body and function with each other form the total organism (one living individual).

I. **MATCHING.**
   Match the correct term to the definition.

1. ___ system		A.	molecules combine together to form this level
2. ___ organism		B.	responsible for all of the movement of the body
3. ___ muscle		C.	protects cavities and organ structures from injury and fluid loss
4. ___ chemical		D.	made up of several organs which have a common function
5. ___ tissue		E.	supports posture and function
6. ___ nervous		F.	made up of groups of cells and the materials surrounding them
7. ___ cellular		G.	tissues combine to form this level
8. ___ connective		H.	largest structural level
9. ___ epithelial		I.	tissue which is the communication system of the body
10. ___ organ		J.	atoms and molecules

Disease Processes

The term *disease* is a generic term which means (as defined by *Dorland's Medical Dictionary*):

"Any deviation from or interruption of the normal structure or function of any part, organ or system (or any combination thereof) of the body manifested by a characteristic set of symptoms and signs, and whose **etiology**, **pathology**, and **prognosis** may be known or unknown."

Highlights

Modern medicine comes down to identifying (diagnosing) the cause of disease (etiology) within the human body and prescribing treatments and therapies to try to fix them.

This definition encompasses virtually everything imaginable that can go wrong with the body. A disease can be a lesion, an injury, an infection, a state or condition—virtually anything, including pregnancy, that is a departure from the norm. (Apparently, not being pregnant is considered the "normal" state of a woman.)

Modern medicine, for all intents and purposes, is simply the identification of disease processes and their treatment. This is true regardless of the type of specialty or nature of the disease.

Disease Classification

Billions of dollars are spent on research to learn more about the etiology (cause) of disease. If modern medicine had a perfect understanding of the etiology of every disease, then treatments, therapies, and interventions could be perfected and quality of life would be vastly improved. In many cases diseases have been eradicated; in many cases understanding has led to better management/therapies but not cures; and, of course, many etiologies are still completely unknown.

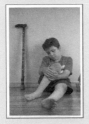

Polio is a contagious disease (virus caused by poliovirus) that wreaked havoc throughout the centuries. In 1952, 58,000 cases were reported in the U.S. with 3,145 deaths and 21,269 left with mild to severe disabling paralysis. In 1789, British physician Michael Underwood described polio as "a debility of the lower extremities." However, ancient Egyptian carvings of otherwise healthy-looking children with canes and withered lower limbs lead many to believe that polio is a virus with pre-history roots. Research and understanding of the mechanism of the polio virus led Jonas Salk to develop a polio vaccine in 1952. Understanding of the etiology of polio with the resultant vaccine administered through a nationwide vaccination program led to the virtual eradication of polio in the United States. Americans were declared "polio free" in 2002 by the World Health Organization.

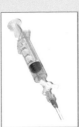

Research into the etiology of the "sugar sickness" led 18th and 19th century medical pioneers like Matthew Dobson, Thomas Willis, John Rollo, Paul Langerhans, and George Zuelzer to make discoveries about the relationships between the pancreas, insulin, diet, blood sugar, and weight. Twentieth century scientists were able to make breakthroughs with Leonard Thompson, age 14, being the first human to receive an insulin injection in 1922. In the early 1920s, Frederick Bantin and Charles Best isolated insulin and eventually won the Nobel Prize. Around 1925, the first home blood sugar testing was developed. Today, people with diabetes can live longer than in the past through management with insulin and other pharmaceuticals, blood sugar testing, and management of diet and exercise. Understanding the etiology of diabetes has advanced rapidly in the last two centuries, and research continues to focus on finding a cure.

One way diseases are classified is by their etiologies. Consider the two diseases showcased above. Polio is introduced into the body from the outside. A person breathes in the polio virus that binds to their cells and causes the person to have polio. A person doesn't "catch" diabetes. Diabetes results from a malfunction of a person's autoimmune system, where the body destroys its own ability to manufacture insulin.

The upcoming lessons will give you some exposure (fortunately not infectious exposure) to disease classifications. As you read each classification, notice that some diseases can be classified in more than one classification.

Disease Classification Terms – Lesson 1

I. TERMINOLOGY.
Enter each term in the space provided. Read the definition and description for each term.

1. **acquired** _____

This means that the patient was not born with it (it was not hereditary or congenital).
Example: AIDS—acquired immunodeficiency syndrome

2. **congenital** _____

Present at birth. This differs from a hereditary condition in that it is not necessarily inherited from the parents. Occasionally infants are born with a congenital heart defect that requires surgery or leads to death.
Example: Congenital hydrocephalus

3. **deficiency** _____

A lack or defect. Many diseases are caused by a lack of some vital chemical substance or compound, such as a lack of red blood cells, defined as anemia or a lack of oxygen, characterizing hypoxia.
Example: Iron deficiency anemia

4. **degenerative** _____

Pertaining to deteriorating. Going from normal to less than normal or dysfunctional. The deterioration of anatomical structures or tissues causes many different diseases, such as degenerative joint disease or Alzheimer disease.
Example: Degenerative joint disease

5. **developmental** _____

A type of disease that occurs as a result of some abnormality in the development of tissue, an organ, or body part. These are often characterized as disorders, and many of them occur before birth or during the growth stages, such as osteodystrophy.
Example: Muscular dystrophy

II. MATCHING.
Match the correct term to the definition.

1. ____ acquired

2. ____ developmental

3. ____ deficiency

4. ____ congenital

5. ____ degenerative

A. deteriorating

B. present at birth

C. lack or defect

D. abnormality in development of tissues or organs

E. not born with it

III. FILL IN THE BLANK.
Use the words in the box to fill in the blanks.

1. Most diseases that afflict people throughout their life are, in fact,
   _____. In other words, they have at some point
   since birth developed the disease.

2. The opposite of an acquired disease, a _____
   disease is present at birth.

3. Severe _____ joint disease of the knees is now
   noted, having worsened significantly over the past five years.

4. Aplasia of the fingers is a _____ anomaly,
   occurring in utero.

5. When the thyroid gland fails to produce enough thyroid
   hormone, this is called hypothyroidism, and is a
   _____ of the thyroid.

developmental
congenital
acquired
degenerative
deficiency

Disease Classification Terms – Lesson 2

I. TERMINOLOGY.
Enter each term in the space provided. Read the definition and description for each term.

1. essential _____

A term assigned to diseases for which the cause is unknown. It is assumed that it arises
spontaneously, such as in essential hypertension.
Example: Essential hypertension

2. familial _____

Occurring in or affecting more members of a family than would be expected by chance alone, such
as familial hypertrophic cardiomyopathy. This would suggest a hereditary component.
Example: Familial hemophagocytic reticulosis

3. functional _____

A functional disease is one in which the structure is unaffected but it is not functioning properly. An
example is menorrhea or menorrhagia that cannot be explained by fibroids, endometriosis, infection,
or some other obvious cause.
Example: Psychogenic disorder

4. **hereditary** _____

This term means genetically transmitted from parent to offspring, and should be a familiar term. As with any trait—eye color, hair color, height, etc.—diseases can be genetically transferred. Examples include hemophilia, dyslexia, and asthma.
Example: Hemophilia

5. **idiopathic** _____

This also means of unknown cause, arising spontaneously, such as idiopathic cardiomyopathy.
Example: Spontaneous pneumothorax

II. MATCHING.
Match the correct term to the definition.

1. ___ functional
2. ___ essential
3. ___ familial
4. ___ idiopathic
5. ___ hereditary

A. suggests a hereditary component
B. transmitted from parent to child
C. of unknown cause
D. normal structure not working properly; no underlying cause
E. of unknown cause or spontaneous origin

III. FILL IN THE BLANK.
Use the words in the box to fill in the blanks.

1. With no obvious origin, he has been diagnosed with

   _____ hypertension.

2. Her daughter has also been diagnosed with _____

   dysautonomia.

3. A _____ disease is diagnosed when there is no

   structural abnormality present.

4. An _____ disease arises spontaneously.

5. Familial is a similar descriptive term for this type of disease.

   _____

| hereditary |
| familial |
| essential |
| functional |
| idiopathic |

Disease Classification Terms – Lesson 3

I. **TERMINOLOGY.**
   Enter each term in the space provided. Read the definition and description for each term.

1. **infectious** _____

   A disease that is caused by an infection (that makes sense, doesn't it?). An infection is the invasion and multiplication of microorganisms in body tissue. There are many different types of bacteria that cause infection and infective diseases, such as pneumonia and mononucleosis. Other infectious agents are viruses and fungi.
   Example: Streptococcal aureus

2. **molecular** _____

   A disease caused by abnormality in the chemical structure or concentration of a single molecule (the smallest amount of a substance which can exist alone), usually a protein or enzyme. Molecular diseases are often also congenital.
   Example: Sickle cell anemia

3. **neoplastic** _____

   Pertaining to any new and abnormal growth, specifically a new growth of tissue which is progressive and uncontrolled. These growths are generally called tumors. A neoplasm can be either benign or malignant. Malignant means tending to become progressively worse, resulting in death. Benign is simply the opposite of malignant. Cancer is an example of a neoplastic disease.
   Example: Malignant neoplasm

4. **nutritional** _____

   A disease caused by nutritional factors, such as insufficient or excessive dietary intake. Common nutritional diseases are eating disorders, such as bulimia or anorexia nervosa. Scurvy is an example of a disease caused by poor nutrition and vitamin deficiency.
   Example: Rickets

5. **organic** _____

   A disease that is due to a demonstrable abnormality in a bodily structure or the composition of its fluids.
   Example: Heart murmur

6. **traumatic** _____

   Resulting from some type of injury: physical, chemical, or psychological. Many pathologies fall into this category, such as fractures, burns, dislocations, cuts, injuries from a motor vehicle or other accidents, war wounds, or the psychological effects of abuse, war, or rape, leading to diseases such as post-traumatic stress disorder.
   Example: Laceration

II. MATCHING.

1. ____ traumatic
2. ____ nutritional
3. ____ neoplastic
4. ____ infectious
5. ____ molecular
6. ____ organic

A. resulting from injury
B. abnormality of a bodily structure
C. related to a tumor
D. caused by dietary intake
E. abnormality of a single molecule
F. caused by infection

III. FILL IN THE BLANK.
Use the words in the box to fill in the blanks.

1. An example of a(n) _____ disease would be gout, historically linked to excessive intake of rich alcoholic drinks and rich or sweet foods.

2. The car accident caused several _____ injuries.

3. A heart murmur is an example of a(n) _____ disease.

4. When a disease is related to a tumor or growth it is considered a(n) _____ disease.

5. Microorganisms invade tissue, creating _____ diseases.

6. An abnormality in a protein or an enzyme is often a(n) _____ disease.

organic
nutritional
neoplastic
molecular
traumatic
infectious

Disease Classification Terms – Lesson 4

The last lesson in this unit introduces you to some classification terms for diseases that, unlike the first three lessons, are not based on disease etiology. Lesson 4 introduces you to some ways of describing (classifying) disease based on patient symptomatology, disease staging, or disease duration.

I. TERMINOLOGY.
Enter each term in the space provided. Read the definition and description for each term.

1. **acute** _____

A short and relatively severe course. A patient with an acute illness has not been experiencing symptoms for very long. An example of this would be acute appendicitis. This is an inflammation of the appendix, which develops quickly and often necessitates surgery because of the severity of the symptoms and the likelihood of the appendix bursting.
Example: Acute respiratory failure

2. **asymptomatic** _____

Having no symptoms. Although generally individuals do not go to a doctor or hospital when they are not experiencing symptoms, underlying asymptomatic diseases are often discovered during examinations, which are either routine or being performed for a different reason.
Example: Asymptomatic human immunodeficiency virus

3. **chronic** _____

Persisting over a long period of time. This is the opposite of acute. A chronic condition can last for months, years, and even a lifetime. One example is chronic bronchitis, which results in daily and sometimes constant coughing and changes in the lung tissue.
Example: Chronic obstructive lung disease

4. **disabling** _____

Causes impairment of normal functions. This could include impairment of motility (walking), breathing, feeding oneself, sight, hearing, standing up, etc.
Example: Blindness

5. **end-stage** _____

A progressively deteriorating condition that has reached a point of terminal functional impairment of the affected organ or system. An example of this is end-stage liver disease, when the liver is so severely affected by incurable cirrhosis that it is in the final phases of ceasing to function.
Example: End stage renal disease

II. MATCHING.
Match the correct term to the definition.

1. ____ acute		A.	impairs normal function
2. ____ chronic		B.	terminal impairment
		C.	persisting for a long time
3. ____ end-stage		D.	short and severe
4. ____ asymptomatic		E.	having no symptoms
5. ____ disabling			

III. FILL IN THE BLANK.
Use the words in the box to fill in the blanks.

1. Death often follows _____ diseases.

2. After being treated for her _____ condition, she still required the use of a wheelchair for mobility.

3. After 24 hours of severe nausea and vomiting, the patient came in for treatment of her _____ condition.

4. _____ bronchitis can cause daily productive cough.

5. Because the foreign object continues to be _____ , no attempts to remove it will be made at this time.

| disabling |
| asymptomatic |
| end-stage |
| acute |
| chronic |

Unit 3
Skeletal System

Skeletal System – Introduction

Your study of Anatomy, Physiology, and Disease Processes began with a high-level description of the structural levels of human anatomy—chemical, cellular, tissue, organ, system, and organism. Building on your understanding of those structural levels, you are going to learn more about each of the body systems that make up the human body. You'll be starting with the skeletal system since the body is built around "Dem Bones!"

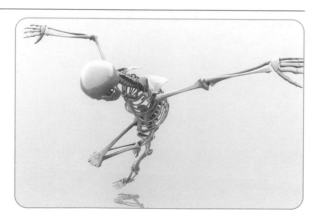

> *With the toe bone connected to the foot bone,*
> *and the foot bone connected to the ankle bone,*
> *and the ankle bone connected to the leg bone.*
> *With the leg bone connected to the knee bone,*
> *and the knee bone connected to the thigh bone,*
> *and the thigh bone connected to the hip bone.*
> *With the hip bone connected to the back bone,*
> *and the back bone connected to the neck bone,*
> *and the neck bone connected to the head bone,*
> *With the finger bone connected to the hand bone,*
> *and the hand bone connected to the arm bone,*
> *and the arm bone connected to the shoulder bone,*
> *With the shoulder bone connected to the back bone,*
> *and the back bone connected to the neck bone,*
> *and the neck bone connected to the head bone.*

Of course, although the song is anatomically correct, there are more technical terms for the skeletal system. In the following unit, we will discuss:

- The purpose, composition, formation, and development of bones.
- The types of bones found in the body.
- The names, locations, and any special markings or purposes for specific bone types.

Axial and Appendicular

The human skeleton is made of densely packaged and calcified connective tissue. At birth, the human body has anywhere from 275–350 bones. As the body matures, some bones in the wrists, ankles, sacrum, coccyx, etc. fuse together, reducing that number to 206 bones. All of these bones working together are classified as the skeletal system.

The bones of the human skeleton are placed into two divisions: the axial skeleton and the appendicular skeleton.

Axial skeleton: The axial skeleton has 80 bones and includes the bones of the skull, vertebral column, thoracic cage, sternum, hyoid, and ears.

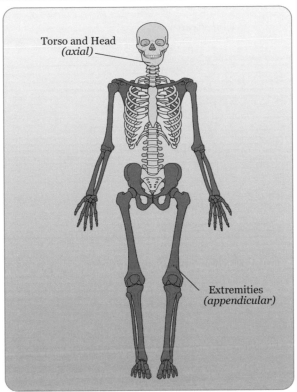

- Skull 27 (8 paired and 5 unpaired cranial and facial bones, including 6 ossicles of the ears)
- Lower Jaw 1
- Hyoid
- Vertebrae 26 bones
- Chest 25 bones
- Total 80

Appendicular skeleton: The appendicular skeleton has 126 bones and includes the bones of the upper and lower extremities.

- Upper extremities 64 bones
- Lower extremities 62 bones
- Total 126

Review: Axial and Appendicular

I. **TERMINOLOGY.**
Enter each term in the space provided. Read the definition and description for each term.

1. **axial skeleton** _____

The 80 bones that comprise the head and trunk.

2. **appendicular skeleton** _____

The 126 bones that comprise the body's upper and lower extremities.

II. MULTIPLE CHOICE.
Choose whether the bone(s) belong to the axial or appendicular skeleton.

1. forearm
   - ○ axial
   - ○ appendicular

2. thighbone
   - ○ axial
   - ○ appendicular

3. skull
   - ○ axial
   - ○ appendicular

4. ossicles (ear bones)
   - ○ axial
   - ○ appendicular

5. calf
   - ○ axial
   - ○ appendicular

6. upper arm
   - ○ axial
   - ○ appendicular

7. vertebrae
   - ○ axial
   - ○ appendicular

8. feet
   - ○ axial
   - ○ appendicular

9. lower jaw
   - ○ axial
   - ○ appendicular

10. neck
    - ○ axial
    - ○ appendicular

11. elbow

○ axial
○ appendicular

12. chest

○ axial
○ appendicular

13. knees

○ axial
○ appendicular

14. ankles

○ axial
○ appendicular

Skeletal Function

The skeleton has multiple functions, three of which are:

- To form the framework of the human body.
- To serve as a means of attachment for muscles.
- To protect vital organs such as the heart, lungs, and brain.

These functions are likely self-explanatory given your personal experience having your own human body. Unlike jellyfish, humans have a solid framework that encases important organs and gives people substance and shape. The skeletal system also has functions that are not so apparent in everyday life (unless they stop working!) but that are equally important:

- Bone marrow and cell formation
- Mineral storage

The internal soft tissues of the bones contain marrow, which is responsible for erythropoiesis (the formation of red blood cells) and the formation of certain white blood cells.

Erythropoietic marrow is found in:

- hip bones
- proximal ends of the thigh and arm bones
- bones of the skull
- vertebrae
- sternum

This erythropoietic marrow is the medium for the development and storage of about 95% of the body's blood cells. Red blood cells and certain white blood cells are formed here, as are stem cells. These cells are very important and serve the following specific functions:

Red blood cells, also called erythrocytes, carry oxygen from the lungs to the rest of the body and return carbon dioxide and other waste products.

White blood cells, also called leukocytes, help fight infections and generally support the immune system.

There are many different types of white blood cells, including:

- lymphocytes
- monocytes
- eosinophils
- basophils
- neutrophils (granulocytes)

All blood cells form from stem cells found in the bone marrow.

Measurement of the body's red blood cells and white blood cells is extremely important in the identification, diagnosis, and treatment of diseases.

Bones also store minerals, such as calcium and phosphorus, which are released into the blood stream as needed. These minerals provide bones with their rigidity and strength. The lack of these minerals or improper absorption by the blood stream can cause a variety of maladies of the skeleton, such as osteoporosis, in which the bones break easily even when there has been minimal trauma.

Review: Function

I. **MULTIPLE CHOICE.**
   Choose the best answer.

1. Erythrocytes
   - ○ red blood cells
   - ○ white blood cells

2. Lymphocytes
   - ○ red blood cells
   - ○ white blood cells

3. Red blood cells
   - ○ carry oxygen from the lungs to the rest of the body
   - ○ help fight infections and aid the immune system
   - ○ reproduce themselves and all other blood cells

4. White blood cells
   - ○ carry oxygen from lungs to rest of body
   - ○ help fight infections and aid the immune system
   - ○ reproduce themselves and all other blood cells

5. Stem cells
   ○ carry oxygen from lungs to rest of body
   ○ help fight infections and aid the immune system
   ○ reproduce themselves and all other blood cells

6. Monocytes
   ○ red blood cells
   ○ white blood cells

7. Neutrophils
   ○ red blood cells
   ○ white blood cells

8. Phosphorus is a _____.
   ○ red blood cell
   ○ white blood cell
   ○ mineral

9. Minerals provide bones with _____.
   ○ marrow
   ○ rigidity and strength
   ○ immunization against infection

Bone Formation and Development

During the eighth week (or so) of development, the human embryo begins the process of ossification (bone formation). This early bone formation produces immature bone, which is rather different from mature bone found in the adult skeleton. Immature bone is similar to bone tissue that forms during repair of bone fractures—it contains many fibers and cells, and less of the cement and mineral substances found in mature bone. Over time, the bulk of immature bone is replaced by mature bone.

Bone is made up of three different cell types: osteoblasts, osteocytes, and osteoclasts.

Highlights

The process of bone formation is called ossification.
Bone is made up of three different cell types:

1. osteoblasts
2. osteocytes
3. osteoclasts

Bone formation (ossification) begins when osteoblasts appear in the body. Osteoblasts secrete an organic matrix into which bone salts are deposited to initiate the process of calcification (hardening). The matrix in which young bone is formed, as well as the young bone itself that is created, is called osteoid. The term *osteoid* also means "resembling bone."

When the osteoblasts are finally surrounded by this matrix, they become osteocytes (former osteoblasts). The purpose of osteocytes is to regulate the increased bone metabolism that occurs with growth and development.

Osteoblasts continue to form immature bone while bone growth and development ensure that immature bone is replaced by mature bone. Replacement occurs when osteoclasts attach themselves to immature bone, dissolve it, and then reabsorb it. Throughout the process, there is a constant turnover of bone matrix, which can result in remodeling of bone.

Two similar forms of ossification, intramembranous and intracartilaginous (endochondral), have the same purpose: to replace membrane and cartilage with bone. Ossification in the human body is completed by about age 25. This continued ossification is the reason why fractures, breaks, or ruptures in bone tissue heal much more easily and with fewer complications in a young person's skeleton than they do in an older person's skeleton.

Term	Definition
bone cells	Cells the body has programmed to create bones
immature bone	The first formation of bone
mature bone	Bone that has ossified and calcified
ossification	Bone formation
osteoblasts	Bone-forming cells that secrete a matrix which becomes calcified
osteoclasts	Large multinucleated cells that reabsorb bone matrix
osteocytes	Former osteoblasts that are surrounded by bone matrix and have calcified

I. **MATCHING.**
   Match the correct term to the definition.

1. ____ bone cells

2. ____ osteoblasts

3. ____ osteocytes

4. ____ immature bone

5. ____ osteoclasts

6. ____ mature bone

7. ____ ossification

A. bone-forming cells that secrete a matrix which becomes calcified

B. former osteoblasts that are surrounded by bone matrix and have calcified

C. large multinucleated cells that reabsorb bone matrix

D. the first formation of bone

E. bone that has ossified and calcified

F. bone formation

G. cells that the body has programmed to create bones

II. FILL IN THE BLANK.
Use the word(s) in the box to fill in the blanks.

1. Bone formation begins when _____ appear in the body.

2. Another term for hardening of bone is _____.

3. _____ is the name of the bone cell that dissolves and reabsorbs immature bone.

4. When osteoblasts are surrounded by matrix they become _____.

5. Another name for white blood cells is _____.

6. Thrombocytes (platelets) help control _____

7. _____ blood cells help fight infection.

8. Another name for erythrocytes is _____ blood cells.

9. Erythropoietic bone marrow is responsible for _____ of the body's blood cells.

10. The legs are part of the _____ skeleton.

11. The jawbone is part of the _____ skeleton.

12. The _____ bone is the only floating bone in the body.

13. Another name for bone formation is _____.

14. Intramembranous and intracartilaginous are two forms of _____.

15. The three basic bone cells are osteoblasts, osteocytes, and _____.

16. _____ is the process in which marrow forms red blood cells, certain white blood cells, and stem cells.

| axial |
| osteoclasts |
| white |
| appendicular |
| osteoblasts |
| erythropoiesis |
| calcification |
| red |
| bleeding |
| osteocytes |
| 95% |
| hyoid |
| osteoclasts |
| ossification |
| leukocytes |
| ossification |

Bone Types

There are two types of bone tissue found in mature bones: cortical (compact) bone and cancellous (spongy) bone.

Cortical Bone

Cortical (compact) bone represents almost 80% of the skeletal mass of the human body. It is called "compact" because it forms a protective outer layer around every bone in the body.

The structural unit of compact bone is the osteon. If you were to examine a cross section of cortical bone, you would see what appears to be groupings of bullseyes.

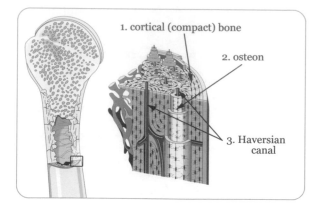

These are osteons. Each osteon has a central canal (Haversian canal) containing capillaries, arterioles, venules, nerves, and probably lymphatics. Between the osteons are interstitial lamellae (3–15 layers of mineralized bone). The overall structural pattern of cortical (compact) bone gives it a plywood-like strength that is highly resistant to bending, torsion, and breakage. Cortical bone has a very slow turnover rate.

Cancellous Bone

Cancellous (spongy) bone represents only about 20% of the skeletal mass, but 80% of bone surface.

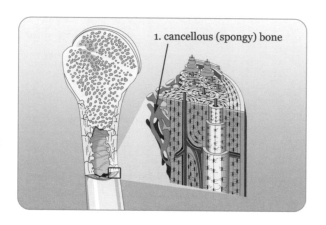

Cancellous bone contains a trabecular (mesh-like) network of bone tissue that allows it to maintain its shape despite compressive forces. The structural unit of cancellous bone has several characteristics: (1) it does not contain osteons; (2) it is less dense than cortical bone; (3) it is very elastic; (4) it has a higher turnover rate than cortical bone. Cancellous bone maintains an intricate balance of bone cells, marrow, and other tissues vital for bone formation. It is as hard as cortical bone, but it is formed in such a way as to appear spongy or mesh-like. Cancellous bone comprises most of the bone in the axial skeleton, including the bones of the skull, ribs, ears, and spine.

As mentioned previously, bone is an intricate and dynamic part of the human body. Not only does bone tissue regulate the production of blood cells, it performs other important functions as well. Bone is not "dead" tissue. An example of its dynamic nature is its ability to heal itself quickly when fractures occur.

Review: Bone Types

I. **TERMINOLOGY.**
   Enter each term in the space provided. Read the definition and description for each term.

   1. **canaliculi** _____

   The narrow channels through which the osteocytes extend.

   2. **cancellous bone** _____

   A spongy structure; refers mostly to bone tissue.

3. **cortical (compact) bone** _____

The hard layer that generally makes up the outer surface of bones.

4. **lacunae** _____

Small cavities containing mature bone cells.

5. **osteocytes** _____

Mature bone cells.

II. MULTIPLE CHOICE.
Choose the best answer.

1. (◯ Lacunae, ◯ Laminae, ◯ Osteocytes) are small cavities of mature bone cells.

2. Bone tissue that is spongy is (◯ cortical, ◯ sesamoid, ◯ cancellous) bone.

3. The outer layer of a bone is called (◯ cancellous, ◯ canaliculi, ◯ compact) bone.

4. (◯ Canaliculi, ◯ Cancellous, ◯ Cortical) are narrow channels of osteocytes.

5. (◯ Osteoblasts, ◯ Osteoclasts, ◯ Osteocytes) are mature bone cells.

6. (◯ Immature bone, ◯ Mature bone, ◯ Marrow) is the spongy substance contained within bones.

7. Osteoclasts dissolve and reabsorb (◯ mature bone, ◯ immature bone, ◯ osteoarthritis).

8. (◯ White blood cells, ◯ Red blood cells, ◯ Stem cells) are produced in bones and help fight infection.

Types of Bones

The human skeleton consists of bones of many different shapes and sizes.

I. TERMINOLOGY.
Enter each term in the space provided. Read the definition and description for each term.

1. **long bones** _____

Long bones are bones whose length is greater than their width, such as the bones of the extremities (tibia, fibula, femur, radius, ulna, humerus).

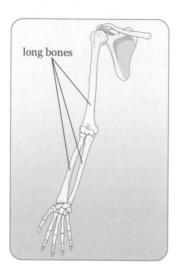

2. **short bones** _____

Short bones are shaped more like cubes and are generally found in the ankle and wrist (carpus and tarsus).

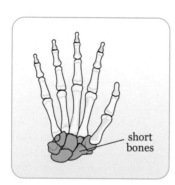

3. **flat bones** _____

Flat bones are found in the cranial vault, sternum (breastbone), shoulder blades, and ribs. Flat bones are made up of a layer of marrow (diploe) sandwiched between two layers of compact bone.

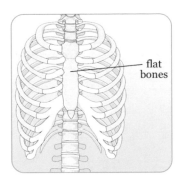

4. **irregular bones** _____

Irregular bones are a mix of irregularly shaped bones that do not fall into any of the other bone-type categories. They are found in the face, spinal column, and hips.

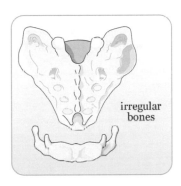

5. **sesamoid bones** _____

Sesamoid bones are mostly rounded masses embedded in certain tendons and are usually related to the surfaces of joints. Included in this group are the patella (kneecap), metacarpophalangeal joints of the hands, and metatarsophalangeal joints of the toes.

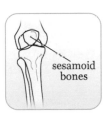

6. **wormian bones** _____

Wormian bones are small bones found between suture lines of the skull where the edges of the skull bones are joined together.

Bone Markings

Besides knowing the types, functions, and shapes of bones, there are also markings that differentiate bones. For example, some bones have parts with a "scooped out" look. Depending on the size of the scooped out area, this feature is known as a fossa, groove, or pit. Other bones have an opening or hole in them referred to as a foramen.

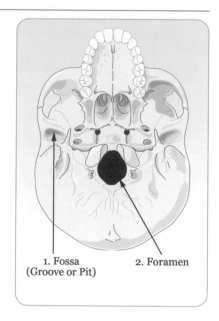

1. Fossa (Groove or Pit) 2. Foramen

I. **TERMINOLOGY.**

   Enter each term in the space provided. Read the definition and description for each term.

   1. **sinuses** _____

   Cavities inside a bone.

   2. **head** _____

   Rounded end of a long bone (the rounded tip).

   3. **foramen** _____

   Opening or hole in a bone.

   4. **tubercle** _____

   Small rounded projections.

   5. **fossa/groove/pit** _____

   Indentation of a bone, also called a depression.

   6. **condyles/epicondyles** _____

   Rounded bone projections.

   7. **neck** _____

   Constricted end of a long bone before the head or rounded end.

   8. **canal/meatus** _____

   Long or deep hole in a bone.

9. **facets** _____

Small, smooth, and flat areas.

10. **tuberosity** _____

Large rounded projections.

II. **MULTIPLE CHOICE.**
   Determine if the following terms are a bone marking or a type of bone.

1. condyles
   - ○ Bone marking
   - ○ Bone type

2. long
   - ○ Bone marking
   - ○ Bone type

3. neck
   - ○ Bone marking
   - ○ Bone typo

4. sinuses
   - ○ Bone marking
   - ○ Bone type

5. short
   - ○ Bone marking
   - ○ Bone type

6. cavity
   - ○ Bone marking
   - ○ Bone type

7. sesamoid
   - ○ Bone marking
   - ○ Bone type

8. wormian
   - ○ Bone marking
   - ○ Bone type

9. facets
- ◯ Bone marking
- ◯ Bone type

10. tubercle
- ◯ Bone marking
- ◯ Bone type

11. irregular
- ◯ Bone marking
- ◯ Bone type

12. tuberosity
- ◯ Bone marking
- ◯ Bone type

13. flat
- ◯ Bone marking
- ◯ Bone type

14. foramen
- ◯ Bone marking
- ◯ Bone type

15. meatus
- ◯ Bone marking
- ◯ Bone type

16. fossa
- ◯ Bone marking
- ◯ Bone type

The Skull and Fontanels

The axial skeletal system consists of, as previously noted, the bones of the skull, vertebral column, thoracic cage, sternum, hyoid, and ears. This creates the structure for most of the vital areas of the body, providing support and protection for the inner organs, as well as movement through the neck and the spine.

Bones of the Skull

There are 27 bones in the skull. The cranium contains 6 main bones, the face has 15 bones, and the ossicles of the ears have 6 bones (3 per ear).

Fontanels

At birth, the bones of the head are not completely formed. As a result, there is adequate space between them to allow the baby's head to be molded enough to fit through the birth canal. These 6 spaces are known as fontanels or "soft spots."

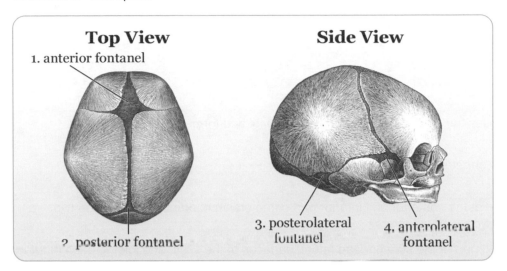

Top View
1. anterior fontanel
2. posterior fontanel

Side View
3. posterolateral fontanel
4. anterolateral fontanel

I. **TERMINOLOGY.**
   Enter each term in the space provided. Read the definition and description for each term.

   1. **anterior fontanel** _____

   The space where the frontal angles of the parietal bones meet the two ununited halves of the frontal bone.

   2. **posterior fontanel** _____

   The space where the occipital angles of the parietal bones meet the occipital.

   3. **anterolateral fontanels** _____

   An interval on either side of the head where the frontal angle of the temporal bone and greater wing of the sphenoid meet.

   4. **posterolateral fontanels** _____

   The interval on either side of the head between the mastoid angle of the parietal bone, the temporal bone, and the occipital bone.

Main Cranial Bones and Sutures

After birth, the bones of the cranium continue to grow until the fontanels are no longer present. The posterior and anterolateral fontanels usually fill in 2–3 months after birth. The posterolateral fontanels usually fill in at the end of the first year. The anterior fontanel (the largest fontanel) usually fills in by the middle of the second year after birth.

Term	Definition
coronal suture	Joins the frontal bone to the two parietal bones
frontal bone	Bone that closes the anterior part of the cranial cavity and forms the skeleton of the forehead
lambdoid suture	Joins the two parietal bones to the occipital bone
occipital bone	Bone situated at the posterior and inferior part of the cranium; articulating with the two parietal and two temporal bones
parietal bones	Bones forming part of the superior and lateral surfaces of the skull, and joining each other in the midline at the sagittal suture
sagittal suture	Joins one parietal bone to the other parietal bone
squamous suture	Joins the parietal bones to the temporal bones
temporal bones	Bones forming part of the lateral surfaces and the base of the skull, and containing the organs of hearing

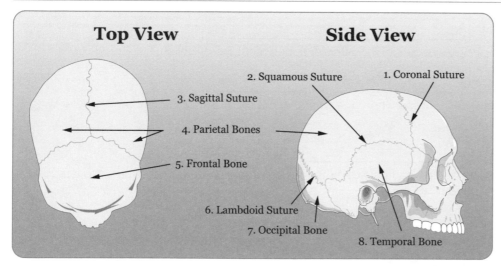

The cranial bones consist of:

- frontal bone
- parietal bones
- occipital bone
- temporal bones

The sutures that join these bones together are:

- coronal suture
- squamous suture
- lambdoid suture
- sagittal suture

I. **TERMINOLOGY.**
   Enter each term in the space provided. Read the definition and description for each term.

   1. **frontal bone** _____

   Bone that closes the anterior part of the cranial cavity and forms the skeleton of the forehead.

   2. **squamous suture** _____

   Joins the parietal bones to the temporal bones.

   3. **parietal bones** _____

   Bones forming part of the superior and lateral surfaces of the skull, and joining each other in the midline at the sagittal suture.

   4. **lambdoid suture** _____

   Joins the two parietal bones to the occipital bone.

   5. **temporal bones** _____

   Bones forming part of the lateral surfaces and the base of the skull, and containing the organs of hearing.

   6. **coronal suture** _____

   Joins the frontal bone to the two parietal bones.

   7. **sagittal suture** _____

   Joins one parietal bone to the other.

   8. **occipital bone** _____

   Bone situated at the posterior and inferior part of the cranium; articulating with the two parietal and two temporal bones.

II. **FILL IN THE BLANK.**
   Looking at the figure further up on this page, please list the names of the cranial bones that are joined by the specified suture. Remember that parietal and temporal bones are bilateral. Bilateral means that there is one on each side (bi = two, lateral = side).

   1. The sagittal suture joins one parietal bone to the other _____ bone.

   2. The squamous sutures join the parietal bones to the _____ bones.

3. The coronal suture joins the _____ bone to the two parietal bones.

4. The lambdoid suture joins the two parietal bones to the _____ bone.

III. **FILL IN THE BLANK.**
Using the words in the box, label the diagram.

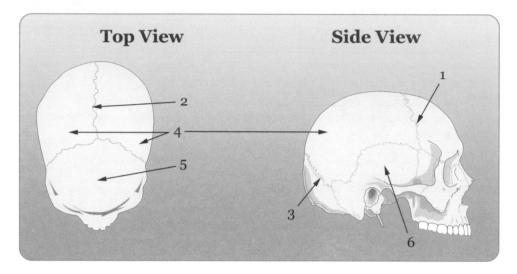

1. _____

2. _____

3. _____

4. _____

5. _____

6. _____

frontal bone
sagittal suture
temporal bone
lambdoid suture
coronal suture
parietal bones

Cranial Bones

The fontanels, sutures, and major cranial bones are only part of the axial skeletal picture. The next several lessons will introduce you to the other axial bones. Let's cover the axial bones from head to toe...well, actually, from head to lower spinal column. The axial bones consist of:

- Bones of the skull
- Ossicles of each ear
- Lower jaw
- Hyoid Bone
- Vertebral column
- Chest

There are 8 sets of paired bones and 5 unpaired bones that make up the bones of the skull.

Paired bones (8 sets for a total of 16):

- nasal concha
- lacrimal bone
- maxilla
- nasal bone
- palatine*
- parietal bone
- temporal bone
- zygomatic bone

Unpaired Bones (5 for a total of 5):

- ethmoid*
- frontal bone
- occipital bone
- sphenoid bone
- vomer

I. **FILL IN THE BLANK.**
   Enter the bolded terms in the space provided.

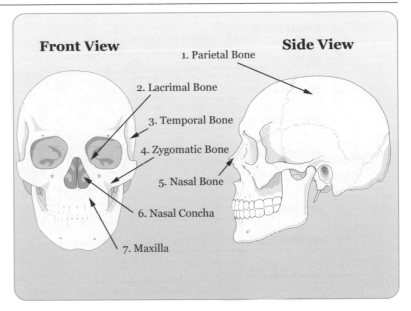

Palatine bone is the bone of the "roof of the mouth" and is not depicted.

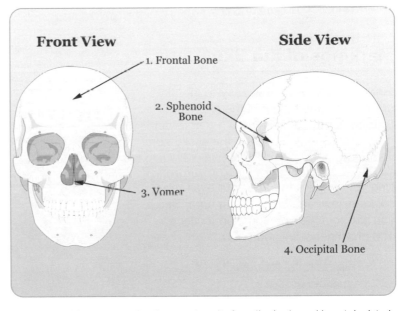

The ethmoid bone separates the nasal cavity from the brain and is not depicted.

Paired bones (8 sets for a total of 16 bones)

1. **nasal concha**_____

2. **lacrimal bone**_____

3. **maxilla**_____

4. **nasal bone**_____

5. **palatine**_____

6. **parietal bone**_____

7. **temporal bone**_____

8. **zygomatic bone**_____

Unpaired Bones (5 bones)

9. **ethmoid**_____

10. **frontal bone**_____

11. **occipital bone**_____

12. **sphenoid bone**_____

13. **vomer**_____

Markings of the Skull

Finally, let's cover a few easy-to-identify markings of the bones of the skull. Remember the definitions of *foramen* and *process*? (Sneak a peek at the sticky note if you forgot.)

Use your fingers to trace your eye sockets, jaw, and behind your ears. See if you can feel the openings, projections, and prominences listed below:

- supraorbital foramen
- mastoid process
- styloid process
- condyloid process
- coronoid process

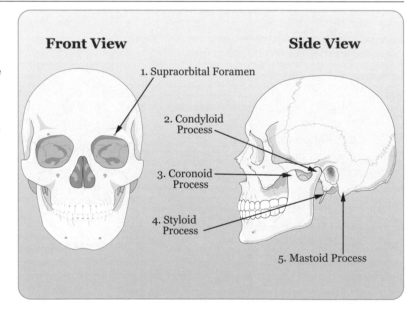

Front View   **Side View**

1. Supraorbital Foramen
2. Condyloid Process
3. Coronoid Process
4. Styloid Process
5. Mastoid Process

Process: prominence or projection, as of bone.

Foramen: opening or hole in a bone.

I. **FILL IN THE BLANK.**
    Enter the bolded word in the blank provided.

1. **supraorbital foramen** _____   2. **mastoid process** _____

3. **styloid process** _____   4. **condyloid process** _____

5. **coronoid process** _____

Ear, Jaw, and Neck Bones

Each ear contains three ossicles. An ossicle is simply a small bone. There are three ossicles per side, for a total of six.

- incus
- malleus
- stapes

The lower jaw contains one bone; this is known as the mandible. The neck contains the only "floating" bone of the entire body. This floating bone, or hyoid bone, is shaped like a U and is supported by the muscles of the neck.

- mandible
- hyoid

I. **FILL IN THE BLANK.**
    Enter the bolded terms in the space provided.

1. **incus** _____

2. **malleus** _____

3. **stapes** _____

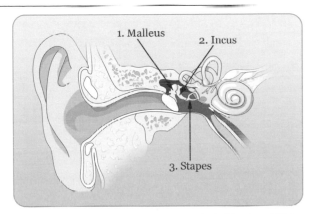

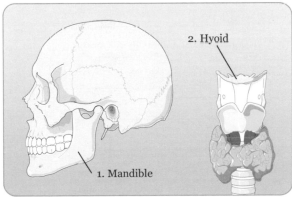

Notice the hyoid bone is at the top of the tracheal tube.

4. mandible _____

5. hyoid _____

Review: The Skull

I. **FILL IN THE BLANK.**
   Use the word(s) in the box to fill in the blanks.

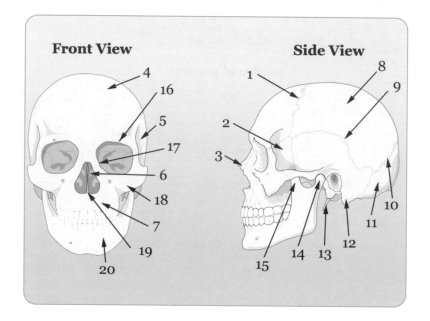

squamous suture	
sphenoid bone	
mandible	
maxilla	
supraorbital foramen	
temporal bone	
coronoid process	
nasal concha	
coronal suture	
mastoid process	
frontal bone	
parietal bone	
condyloid process	
lambdoid suture	
nasal bone	
zygomatic bone	
occipital bone	
vomer	
styloid process	
lacrimal bone	

1. _____

2. _____

3. _____

4. _____

5. _____

6. _____

7. _____

8. _____

9. _____

10. _____

11. _____

12. _____

13. _____

14. _____

15. _____

16. _____

17. _____

18. _____

19. _____

20. _____

II. FILL IN THE BLANK.
Enter the bolded terms in the spaces provided.

1. The **ethmoid** _____ bone is part of the skull and literally means "sieve-like."

2. The occiput gives rise to the **occipital** _____ bone and is the posterior part of the head.

3. The term **nasal** _____ denotes a relationship to the nose.

4. **Concha** _____ means literally "a shell" and is used to describe structures that are shell-like in shape.

5. **Zygomatic** _____ can describe a process, a bone, or an arch.

6. A **foramen** _____ is a natural opening or passage.

7. The upper jaw is made up of the **maxilla** _____ .

8. Shaped like the Greek letter lambda is the **lambdoid** _____ suture.

9. **Condyloid** _____ means resembling a knuckle or rounded bone.

Vertebral Column

The vertebral column consists of 26 total bones, differentiated below. The last lumbar vertebra connects to the sacrum, which connects to the coccyx (or tailbone).

- cervical vertebrae (7)
- atlas vertebra (the first cervical vertebra)
- axis vertebra (the second cervical vertebra)
- thoracic vertebrae (12)
- lumbar vertebrae (5)
- sacrum
- coccyx

The vertebral column is a major support structure for the human body. It consists of 26 bones that are all superimposed on one another, but separated by intervertebral discs. A designated space for passage of the spinal cord runs through the vertebral column housing the core of the central nervous system. In other words, the spinal cord runs right through the center of the bony vertebral column, protecting it from injury.

The vertebral column is not straight like a stack of checkers. The spine has a curvature with portions being convex (rounded like the outside of a sphere) and others being concave (rounded, depressed like the hollowed inner surface of a sphere).

The vertebral column has many other bones and processes that protect and assist in the function of the spine. These will be detailed in future sections.

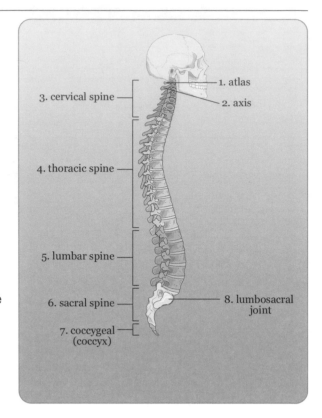

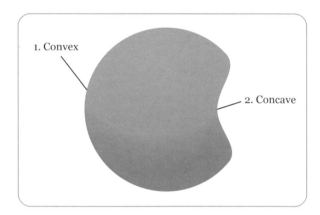

I. TERMINOLOGY.
Enter each term in the space provided. Read the definition and description for each term.

1. **cervical spine** _____

The cervical spine contains 7 vertebrae located in the neck area. In medical reports this spine is abbreviated C1-C7. The cervical spine curve is concave. With the ability to raise the head and stand with erect posture comes the development of this curve, which is why infants are not born with the cervical spine curve.

2. **thoracic spine** _____

The thoracic spine contains 12 vertebrae located in the chest area, which connect to the ribs. In medical reports this spine is abbreviated T1-T12. The thoracic spine curve is convex and is already formed at the time of birth.

3. **articulate** _____

Loosely connect or join. The 12 vertebrae of the thoracic spine articulate to the 12 ribs to form protection for the thoracic cavity.

4. **lumbar spine** _____

The lumbar spine contains 5 vertebrae located in the lower back. The lumbar spine curve is concave. Like the thoracic spine, it is already formed at the time of birth.

5. **sacral spine** _____

The sacral spine consists of 5 fused sacral vertebrae. It is easily distinguishable as an upside-down triangular shape. The two lateral surfaces (sides) are smooth for articulation (loose connection) with the iliac bones of the pelvis.

6. **coccyx (coccygeal spine)** _____

The coccyx or "tailbone" is a single bone formed by fusion of 4-5 coccygeal vertebrae. When pressure is placed on the coccyx, it moves forward and acts like a shock absorber. Sitting down or falling on it too hard can cause it to become fractured. The adjectival form of coccyx is coccygeal.

7. **intervertebral discs** _____

Intervertebral disks (also correctly spelled discs) are composed of fibrous tissue and cartilage located between the vertebrae. Their function is to form strong joints and absorb spinal compression and shock.

II. MATCHING.
Match the correct term to the definition.

1. ____ lumbar spine
2. ____ intervertebral discs
3. ____ cervical spine
4. ____ thoracic spine
5. ____ articulate
6. ____ sacral spine
7. ____ coccyx

A. triangular shaped
B. the neck
C. tailbone
D. join
E. connects to the ribs
F. between the bones of the spine
G. lower back

III. FILL IN THE BLANK.
Use the word(s) in the box to fill in the blanks.

1. Consisting of five vertebrae, the _____ is the lower back.

2. _____ means loosely connect.

3. Consisting of seven vertebrae, the _____ makes up the bones of the neck.

4. Five fused vertebrae make up the _____.

5. The _____ corresponds to the chest cavity and consists of 12 vertebrae.

6. The _____ is also called the tailbone.

7. The spine is made up of several discs; the cartilage and fibrous tissue between them are called _____.

thoracic spine
lumbar spine
intervertebral discs
articulate
coccyx
sacral spine
cervical spine

Sternum and Ribs

The last sections of the axial skeleton to be covered are the sternum and ribs. This portion of the axial skeleton contains:

12 ribs

- true ribs (1–7)
- false ribs (8–10)
- floating (false) ribs (11–12)

sternum

- manubrium
- body
- xiphoid process

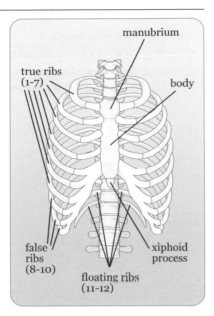

There are 12 pairs of ribs in the human body. These are long, curved bones that attach posteriorly to the thoracic vertebrae. Anteriorly rib pairs 1–7 connect to the sternum and are called true ribs. Ribs 8–10 connect to cartilage anteriorly and are called false ribs. The remaining two ribs, 11–12, are also connected to the thoracic spine posteriorly, but are free from connection anteriorly. Although ribs 11–12 are technically considered false ribs, they are also called floating ribs.

The sternum (breastbone) is a dagger-shaped bone located anteriorly in the middle of the chest. It has three divisions: the upper portion is the manubrium (handle); the middle section (which is the longest part) is the body; and the smallest, most distal portion (i.e., farthest from the handle) is the xiphoid process. The xiphoid process does not ossify until adulthood.

The area on the sternum where the manubrium and the body join is a significant landmark of the chest. It is called the sternal angle.

I. **TERMINOLOGY.**
    Enter each term in the space provided. Read the definition and description for each term.

    1. manubrium _____
    Upper portion (handle) of the sternum.

    2. **body** _____
    Middle section of the sternum.

    3. **xiphoid process** _____
    Distal portion of the sternum.

    4. **sternal angle** _____
    Area of sternum where the manubrium and body join.

Review: Axial Skeleton

I. **FILL IN THE BLANK**
It is important to recall the ability to combine terms as you learned in the Medical Word Building unit. Some answers may require more than one word to be complete. Use the word(s) in the box to fill in the blanks.

1. The uppermost (neck) portion of the vertebral column is the
   _____ spine.

2. The lowermost portion of the spine (joined to the ilium) is the
   _____ spine.

3. The lumbar spine joins with the lowermost portion of the spine.
   Together, these create the _____ junction.

4. The two middle portions of the spine, studied together, are the
   _____ spine.

5. The spine that corresponds to the chest is the
   _____ spine.

6. The shock absorbers of the spinal column are the
   _____.

7. Another name for the tailbone is _____.

8. The curve of the _____ spine does not form until
   the head can be raised and the body stands erect.

9. The sternum is easily identifiable because it is shaped like a
   _____.

10. Because false ribs 11-12 are connected only to the thoracic
    spine, they are also called _____ ribs.

11. The sternal angle is a very significant landmark of the chest and
    is located on the sternum at the junction of the
    _____ and the body.

12. The _____, a part of the sternum, does not ossify
    until adulthood.

13. The vertebral foramen is the area of the spine where the
    _____ passes through.

floating
xiphoid process
cervical
sacral
cervical
spinal cord
thoracic
manubrium
lumbosacral
intervertebral discs
dagger
coccyx
thoracolumbar

Choose the best answer. Some answers may be used more than once, or not at all.

1. ___ lower jaw	A. 26 bones
2. ___ skull	B. 27 bones
3. ___ vertebrae	C. 6 bones
4. ___ chest	D. 25 bones
5. ___ ossicles of ears	E. 1 bone
6. ___ neck	F. 7 bones

Appendicular Skeleton

The appendicular skeleton, as shown to the right, gets its name from the fact that it consists of all the parts that append (hang on) to the axial skeleton. In fact, the arms and legs are known as the appendages.

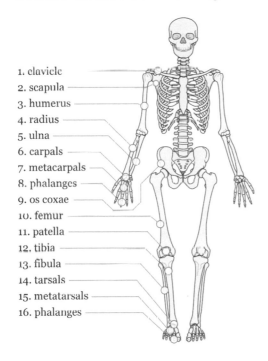

1. clavicle
2. scapula
3. humerus
4. radius
5. ulna
6. carpals
7. metacarpals
8. phalanges
9. os coxae
10. femur
11. patella
12. tibia
13. fibula
14. tarsals
15. metatarsals
16. phalanges

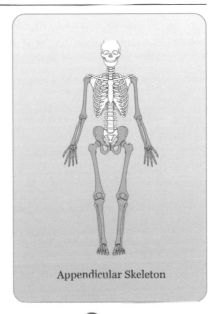

Appendicular Skeleton

You may find it helpful to review terminology like anterior, distal, lateral, inferior, posterior, superior, and medial, as these terms are often used in anatomy for orientation.

In addition to the now-familiar bones of the axial skeleton, the human skeleton has appendicular bones of many shapes and sizes. Take a few minutes to study the bones of the appendicular skeleton.

I. **FILL IN THE BLANK.**
   Please review the following information. Fill in the blanks with the bolded words.

   1. **clavicle** (collarbone) (1 per side for a total of 2) _____

   2. **scapula** (shoulder blade) (1 per side for a total of 2) _____

   3. **humerus** (upper arm) (1 per side for a total of 2) _____

   4. **radius** (forearm) (1 per side for a total of 2) _____

   5. **ulna** (forearm) (1 per side for a total of 2) _____

   6. **carpal** (wrist) (8 per side for a total of 16) _____

   7. **metacarpal** (hand) (5 per side for a total of 10) _____

   8. **phalanges** (fingers) (14 per side for a total of 28) _____

   9. **os coxae** (hip/pelvic bone) (1 per side for a total of 2) _____

   10. **femur** (thigh) (1 per side for a total of 2) _____

   11. **patella** (kneecap) (1 per side for a total of 2) _____

   12. **tibia** (leg) (1 per side for a total of 2) _____

   13. **fibula** (leg) (1 per side for a total of 2) _____

   14. **tarsal** (ankle) (7 per side for a total of 14) _____

   15. **metatarsal** (foot) (5 per side for a total of 10) _____

   16. **phalanges** (toes) (14 per side for a total of 28) _____

Shoulder Bones

Clavicle

The clavicle, or collarbone, is shaped like a loose S and allows the arm to move freely by holding the corresponding shoulder away from the chest. It is the first bone of the human body to ossify. The clavicle is comprised of cancellous bone covered by cortical bone with no bone marrow. The medial or sternal end is attached to the sternum, and the lateral or acromial end is attached to the acromion of the scapula.

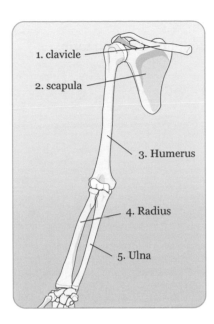

Scapula

The scapula, or shoulder blade, is positioned over ribs 2–7 and lies against the posterior aspect of the ribcage. There are several prominent parts to the scapula: the spine, a long projection that extends to the acromion process to form the point of the shoulder; the coracoid process; and the glenoid cavity, where the head of the humerus rests.

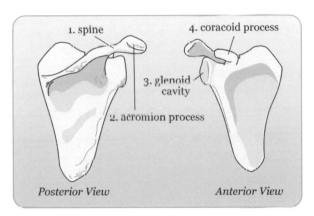

Humerus

The humerus is the upper arm bone. It is a long bone with two ends. The superior end, or the head, is the rounded end and connects to the glenoid cavity of the scapula to form the shoulder joint. This is a ball and socket joint. Below the head is the anatomical neck, which has a small groove/indentation located just beneath the head. Below the anatomical neck is the surgical neck, then the long shaft of the humerus, and finally the inferior end of the bone. The inferior end has lateral and medial epicondyles that are insertion points for muscles of the forearm. An easy way to distinguish the humerus from the femur is to remember that it is not very humorous to "hit" your funny bone (which presses on a nerve near the elbow, causing intense pain).

I. TERMINOLOGY.
Enter each term in the space provided. Read the definition and description for each term.

1. **clavicle** _____
The collarbone; the first bone in the human body to ossify.

2. **sternal end** _____
The end of the clavicle that is attached to the sternum.

3. **acromial end** _____
The end of the clavicle that is attached to the acromion.

4. **scapula** _____
Another name for the shoulder blade.

5. **acromion** _____
Process that helps form point of the shoulder.

6. **coracoid** _____
Process that helps form point of the shoulder.

7. **glenoid cavity** _____
Cavity where the humerus rests.

8. **humerus** _____
Upper arm bone.

II. MATCHING.
Match the correct term to the definition.

1. ____ clavicle
2. ____ glenoid cavity
3. ____ humerus
4. ____ scapula
5. ____ sternal end

A. upper arm bone
B. collar bone
C. medial end
D. where the head of the humerus rests
E. shoulder blade

III. MULTIPLE CHOICE.
   Choose the best answer.

1. The humerus is a_____.
   - ○ long bone
   - ○ short bone
   - ○ wormian bone
   - ○ irregular bone

2. The clavicle is shaped like the letter _____.
   - ○ A
   - ○ N
   - ○ S
   - ○ X

3. The upper arm bone is called the _____.
   - ○ humerus
   - ○ femur
   - ○ scapula
   - ○ clavicle

4. Which of the following is NOT related to the scapula?
   - ○ glenoid cavity
   - ○ acromion
   - ○ epicondyle
   - ○ coracoid

5. Which bone lies against the rib cage, between ribs 2 and 7?
   - ○ clavicle
   - ○ scapula
   - ○ humerus
   - ○ acromion

Arm Bones

The forearm is made up of two separate bones known as the **radius** and the **ulna**.

The radius is one of two bones of the forearm. It is located on the thumb side of the forearm. It has a flattened head at the superior portion where it articulates with the humerus. Further down, below the neck of the radius, is a tuberosity or prominence that is the insertion site for the tendons of the biceps. At the inferior end lies the styloid process for articulation to the carpals. It forms a margin for the tendons of two muscles to the thumb.

Highlights

In anatomy and physiology, articulation is the place of junction between two different parts or objects. *Trochlea* is a general term for a pulley-shaped part or structure.

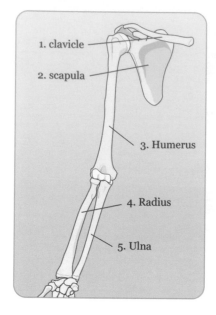

1. clavicle
2. scapula
3. Humerus
4. Radius
5. Ulna

The ulna is the other bone of the forearm and is located on the little finger side. The proximal end of the ulna connects to the elbow to form the elbow joint. Although the radius also articulates with the elbow, the ulna has a stronger connection. Other parts of the ulna include the olecranon, which forms the point of the elbow; the trochlear notch; the coronoid process; the radial notch, where the ulna and radius articulate; the head, which articulates with the wrist and hand; and the styloid process, a bony prominence that can be palpated on the ulnar aspect of the wrist when the hand is palm down.

Take a few minutes to feel the olecranon by bending your elbow and using your fingers to find the "point". Then, putting your palm down, run your fingers along the ulnar (outer) aspect of your wrist. Do you feel the styloid process? Study the graphic of the radius and ulna. Do you see where the ulnar and radius articulate (join) at the radial notch? Can you identify the head, where the radius articulates with the wrist and hand? Finally, think about the definition of *trochlea* (see the highlight box) as you flex and extend your elbow. In addition to the elbow (trochlear notch), where else might your body have pulley-shaped parts or structures? There is a fibrocartilaginous pulley in the frontal bone through which passes the tendon that controls the movement of the superior oblique eye muscle, known as the trochlea musculi olbiqui, superioris oculi. You used an ocular pulley system to read this!

I. TERMINOLOGY.
Enter each term in the space provided. Read the definition and description for each term.

1. **styloid process** _____

Forms a margin for the tendons of two muscles to the thumb.

2. **ulna** _____

Forearm bone located on the pinky side.

3. **olecranon** _____

The large process at the proximal end of the ulna which projects behind the articulation with the humerus and forms the bony prominence of the elbow.

4. **trochlear notch** _____

Pulley-shaped structure of the elbow.

5. **radial notch** _____

Point at which the radius and ulna articulate.

II. MATCHING.
Match the correct term to the definition.

1. ____ ulna
2. ____ tuberosity
3. ____ olecranon
4. ____ radial notch
5. ____ radius

A. thumb-side bone
B. pinky-side bone
C. point of the elbow
D. joint of ulna and radius
E. prominence

III. MULTIPLE CHOICE.
Choose the best answer.

1. The forearm bone closest to the pinky.
   - ○ ulna
   - ○ radius

2. The forearm bone closest to the thumb.
   - ○ ulna
   - ○ radius

3. Which of the following is not part of the ulna?
   - ○ coronoid process
   - ○ olecranon
   - ○ malleolus
   - ○ styloid process

4. A bony prominence.
   - ○ ulna
   - ○ tuberosity
   - ○ radial notch

5. Allows articulation with the carpals.
   - ○ olecranon
   - ○ styloid process

Hand and Wrist Bones

Human wrists, hands, and fingers have incredible dexterity and range of motion. The fine motor ability of the human hand is due, in large part, to the framework of bones with their many muscle and tendon attachments.

- carpals
- metacarpals
- phalanges

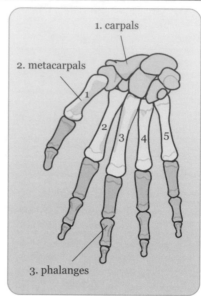

The carpals are the wrist bones. They articulate with the ulna. Carpals are generally made up of 2 rows of 4 bones each and are held in place by ligaments. The 8 carpal bones are the hamate, scaphoid, trapezium, pisiform, trapezoid, lunate, triquetrum, and capitate bones.

The metacarpal bones are the bones of the hands. They consist of 5 bones that form the structure of the hand and articulate with the carpals. These metacarpals are numbered from 1–5, with the thumb being first and the little finger fifth.

The phalanges articulate with the metacarpals to form the fingers. There are 5 fingers, and each has 3 phalanges (the distal, medial, and proximal phalanges), with the exception of the thumb, which has only 2.

I. **TERMINOLOGY.**
    Enter each term in the space provided. Read the definition and description for each term.

    1. **carpals** _____
    Wrist bones.

    2. **metacarpals** _____
    Bones of the hands.

II. **FILL IN THE BLANK.**
    Enter the word in the blank provided.

    1. hamate _____   2. scaphoid _____

    3. trapezium _____   4. pisiform _____

    5. trapezoid _____   6. lunate _____

    7. triquetrum _____   8. capitate _____

1. ____ carpals

2. ____ metacarpals

3. ____ phalanges

A. hands
B. fingers
C. wrists

Hip Bones and Femur

Os Coxae

The hip bone is also called the os coxae. If you view the pelvic girdle anteriorly, it resembles the mask of a superhero. It looks like a hat with wings sitting on top of a mask to cover the eyes. The wings form the ilium, the top of which is the iliac crest. The part of the mask that goes over the eyebrows is formed by the pubic bones. The lower part of the eye mask is formed by the ischium bones, and the portion between the eyes is the symphysis pubis. This lies on the pubic arch. Just think of a superhero when trying to remember the bones of the pelvis.

To support childbearing, the female pelvis is larger than the male pelvis. Unlike the male pelvic structure, the female pelvis has a wide subpubic arch and a forward tilt; the ischial bones are turned outwards and the symphysis pubis is shallow. In addition, the bones of the female pelvis are thin.

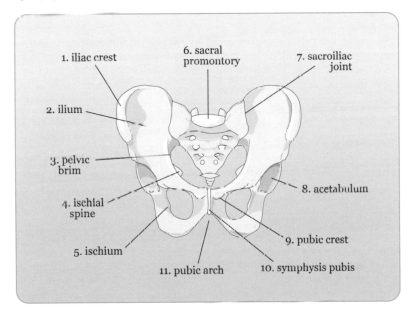

1. iliac crest
2. ilium
3. pelvic brim
4. ischial spine
5. ischium
6. sacral promontory
7. sacroiliac joint
8. acetabulum
9. pubic crest
10. symphysis pubis
11. pubic arch

Highlights

Remember sound alike terms from medical terminology? Note the bone of the hip (spelled I-L-I-U-M). There is an organ of the gastrointestinal system called the ileum (spelled I-L-E-U-M). If you know that I-um is in the hip and E (eat)-um is next to the stomach, it can save you precious time spent looking in a medical dictionary.

Femur

The femur (thigh bone) is the longest and strongest bone in the body. It articulates with the pelvis and two smaller leg bones to form the thigh. At its most superior point the femur consists of a head, neck, greater trochanter, and lesser trochanter. The head of the femur is knob-like and fits perfectly into the acetabulum of the os coxae (to form a ball and socket joint). The greater and lesser trochanters are bony prominences where muscles attach.

The long middle section of the femur is a rounded shaft. At the most inferior end of the shaft are two protrusions (to which ligaments and tendons attach) called the medial epicondyle and the lateral epicondyle. Situated between these two epicondyles is the patellar surface, where the patella or kneecap connects.

A good way to visualize the femur is to think of it as an old-fashioned Barbie doll leg. When Barbie's leg would come off, you had to pop the head of the "femur" back into the hip.

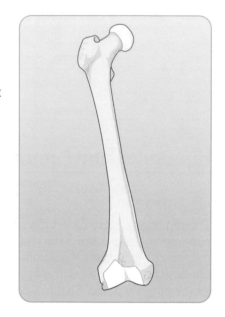

I. TERMINOLOGY.
   Enter each term in the space provided. Read the definition and description for each term.

1. **os coxae** _____
   the hip bone

2. **femur** _____
   the thigh bone

3. **ilium** _____
   wings of the hip bone

4. **ischium** _____
   lower part of the "eye mask" of the hip bone

5. **symphysis pubis** _____
   the portion of the hip bone between the "eyes"

6. **greater trochanter** _____
   bony prominence where muscles attach to the femur

7. **lesser trochanter** _____
   bony prominence where muscles attach to the femur

8. **acetabulum** _____
   a groove in the hip bone

9. **medial epicondyle** _____
   a protrusion to which ligaments and tendons attach on the inferior end of the rounded shaft of the femur

10. **lateral epicondyle** _____

a protrusion to which ligaments and tendons attach on the inferior end of the rounded shaft of the femur

11. **patella** _____

the kneecap

II. MATCHING.
Match the correct term to the definition.

1. ____ femur

2. ____ ischium

3. ____ acetabulum

4. ____ os coxae

5. ____ patella

A. kneecap

B. thigh bone

C. the head of the femur fits into this

D. lower part of the "eye mask"

E. hip bone

III. MULTIPLE CHOICE.
Choose the best answer.

1. The superior portion of the femur consists of all but which ONE of the following?

   ◯ neck
   ◯ greater trochanter
   ◯ lesser trochanter
   ◯ ischium

2. Which of the following is NOT part of the hip bones?

   ◯ os coxae
   ◯ trochanter
   ◯ ilium
   ◯ symphysis pubis

3. The socket portion of the femur ball-and-socket joint.

   ◯ acetabulum
   ◯ patella
   ◯ ischium
   ◯ os coxae

4. Protrusions at the inferior end of the femur.

   ◯ medial and lateral trochanters
   ◯ medial and lateral epicondyles
   ◯ greater and lesser trochanters
   ◯ greater and lesser epicondyles

5. Thigh bone.

   ◯ os coxae
   ◯ patella
   ◯ femur

Lower Leg and Foot Bones

The lower legs, ankle, feet, and toes are the last part of the lower extremities. Like the hands and fingers, there are many small bones that allow mobility and flexibility. Running, jumping, climbing, and walking are made possible by the amazing lower extremity bone structure.

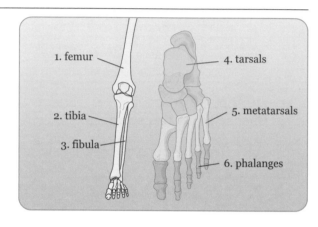

Tibia

The tibia is the largest of the two lower leg bones. It connects with the femur to form the knee joint and is located on the medial (or big toe) side of the leg. The tibia has a sharp, bony ridge that runs lengthwise down the center of the shaft to form the shinbone (which can be felt through the skin on the front of the leg). The most distal point on the medial side of the tibia has a bony extension that is called the medial malleolus (or ankle bone). This protrudes sharply and can be felt on the inner side of the foot. The tibia is the weight-bearing bone of the lower leg.

Fibula

The fibula is a long, skinny lower leg bone that looks rather fragile. It is situated on the lateral (or little toe) side of the leg. It is not a weight-bearing bone. The superior end of the fibula forms the lateral part of the knee joint, and the lateral malleolus forms and protects the lateral portion of the ankle.

Tarsals, Metatarsals, and Phalanges

The tarsals are ankle bones and, along with the other bones in the foot (the metatarsals and phalanges), support weight and act as shock absorbers for the body. There are 7 tarsal bones in each foot: the talus, calcaneus, cuboid, navicular, and 1st, 2nd, and 3rd cuneiforms. The talus articulates with the tibia to bear weight from the legs. The medial malleolus (on the tibia) and the lateral malleolus (on the fibula) protect the talus on both sides.

The metatarsals are the bones of the feet and sit upon arches. There are 5 metatarsals in each foot.

The phalanges or toes connect to the metatarsals. There are 14 phalanges per foot—2 in the great toe and 3 each in the remaining toes. The separations between the phalanges are identified as follows: the distal phalanx (tip of the toe), the middle phalanx, (in the middle) and the proximal phalanx (nearest the point of connection to the metatarsals). Notice that the medical term for toes is the same as for fingers.

I. TERMINOLOGY.
Enter each term in the space provided. Read the definition and description for each term.

1. **tibia** _____
largest of the two lower leg bones

2. **malleolus** _____
the ankle bone that is a bony extension of the tibia

3. **fibula** _____
long, skinny lower leg bone

4. **tarsals** _____
ankle bones that support weight and act as shock absorbers

5. **talus** _____
one of the 7 tarsal bones

6. **calcaneus** _____
one of the 7 tarsal bones

7. **cuboid** _____
one of the 7 tarsal bones

8. **navicular** _____
one of the 7 tarsal bones

9. **cuneiforms** _____
one of the 7 tarsal bones; there are three

10. **metatarsals** _____
bones of the feet that sit upon arches; there are 5 in each foot

11. **phalanges** _____
the toe bones; 14 per foot

II. MATCHING.
Match the correct term to the definition.

1. ____ metatarsals   A. ankle bone(s)

2. ____ tarsals   B. feet bones

     C. larger lower leg bone

3. ____ phalanges   D. toes

4. ____ malleolus   E. protects the ankle

5. ____ tibia

III. MULTIPLE CHOICE.
Choose the best answer.

1. How many phalanges are in the foot?
   - ◯ 3
   - ◯ 6
   - ◯ 14
   - ◯ 9

2. The more fragile of the lower leg bones.
   - ◯ tibia
   - ◯ fibula

3. The stronger and bigger of the lower leg bones.
   - ◯ tibia
   - ◯ fibula

4. Which is not a tarsal bone?
   - ◯ 2nd cuneiform
   - ◯ talus
   - ◯ navicular
   - ◯ epicondyle

5. The primary weight-bearing bone of the leg.
   - ◯ tibia
   - ◯ fibula

Arches of the Foot

A segmented structure like the foot can support weight only if it is arched. Each foot has three arches: the transverse arch, the medial longitudinal arch, and the lateral longitudinal arch. These three arches maintain their strength and flexibility because of the shapes and interlocking capabilities of the bones, ligaments, and tendons of the foot and ankle.

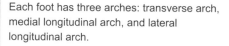

Highlights

Each foot has three arches: transverse arch, medial longitudinal arch, and lateral longitudinal arch.

Arches flex when bearing weight, then return to their normal shape when weight is lifted. The lateral longitudinal arch is a very low arch, arching just enough to redistribute some body weight to the calcaneus and the head of the fifth metatarsal. The medial longitudinal arch is the predominant arch in the foot. It runs from the base of the calcaneus up to the talus, and down again to the three medial metatarsals. (Note: The lateral longitudinal arch extends under the two most lateral metatarsals, and the medial arch extends under the three other metatarsals.)

The above two arches create a frame for the transverse arch, which is formed at the base of the metatarsals (between the tarsals and the metatarsals) and extends from the medial to the lateral sides of the foot. These three arches are shaped such that they are able to distribute the weight of the human body in a 50/50 ratio: half the weight is on the calcaneal bones, and the other half is on the metatarsals; this provides proper balance.

58

The calcaneus (heel bone) is the strongest bone in the foot. It forms the outer part of the ankle and extends back to form the heel. It acts as a shock absorber and bears the immediate stress placed on the foot while walking.

I. TERMINOLOGY.
Enter each term in the space provided. Read the definition and description for each term.

1. **transverse arch** _____

Formed at the base of the metatarsals, extending from the medial to the lateral sides of the foot

2. **medial longitudinal arch** _____

Predominant arch, running from the base of the calcaneus to the talus, and down to the three medial metatarsals

3. **lateral longitudinal arch** _____

Arches just enough to redistribute body weight to the calcaneus and head of the fifth metatarsal

4. **calcaneus** _____ _____

Heel bone; the strongest bone in the foot

Review: Appendicular Skeleton

I. **FILL IN THE BLANK.**

In the blanks provided below, refer to the image and enter the correct term corresponding to the following numbers. Use the word(s) in the box to fill in the blanks.

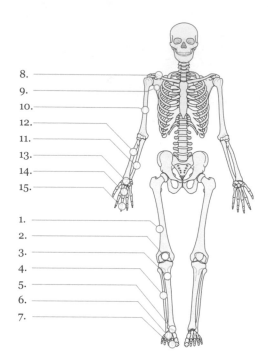

1. _____

2. _____

3. _____

4. _____

5. _____

6. _____

7. _____

8. _____

9. _____

10. _____

11. _____

12. _____

metatarsals
phalanges
clavicle
patella
carpals
scapula
metacarpals
tarsals
humerus
femur
radius
fibula
ulna
tibia

13. _____

14. _____

15. _____

II. FILL IN THE BLANK.
Use the word(s) in the box to fill in the blanks.

1. The bone that runs between the two sets of ribs is the

   _____.

2. Three sets of bones of the pelvis include the pubis, ilium, and

   _____.

3. The three sets of bones that make up the ankles/feet are the

   tarsals, _____, and phalanges.

4. Four bones make up the leg: the femur, _____,

   tibia, and the patella.

5. The shoulder consists of the _____ and the

   clavicle.

6. The bones that hold up the head are the _____.

7. The sternum divides the _____.

8. The main bone of the upper arm is the _____.

9. The two bones of the forearm are the _____ and

   the radius.

10. The name of the head bone is the _____ or skull.

11. The bones of the wrist and hand are the carpals,

    _____, and phalanges.

12. Name the three parts of the phalanges of the feet: distal

    phalanx, medial phalanx, and _____ phalanx.

13. The two sections of the spine that are naturally fused together

    are the sacrum and the _____.

calcaneal
vertebrae
proximal
humerus
metatarsals
femur
cranium
lateral malleolus
scapula
humerus
metacarpals
transverse arch
coccyx
ischium
sternum
tibia
ulna
fibula
ribs
ischium

14. The _____ bone is the strongest bone in the human body.

15. The strongest bone in the foot is the _____ bone.

16. The _____ bone is the bone of the upper arm and the femur bone is the bone of the thigh.

17. The sides of the ankle bones that extend from the leg bones are the medial malleolus and the _____.

18. The three main bones that form the base (superhero mask) of the pelvis are the suprapubic arch, _____, and pubis.

19. The _____ bone is the weight-bearing bone of the lower leg.

20. The three arches of the foot are the medial longitudinal arch, lateral longitudinal arch, and _____.

III. MATCHING.
Match the correct term to the definition.

1. ____ clavicle
2. ____ femur
3. ____ scapula
4. ____ os coxae
5. ____ phalanges
6. ____ humerus
7. ____ carpals
8. ____ tarsals
9. ____ patella
10. ____ tibia

A. wrist bones
B. ankle bones
C. hip bone
D. shoulder blade
E. kneecap
F. strongest bone of the body
G. fingers and toes
H. collarbone
I. upper arm bone
J. weight-bearing bone of the legs

Joints and Articulations

Term	Definition	Example
fibrous joints	No joint cavity and, in general, do not move.	radioulnar and tibiofibular joints
cartilaginous joints	Have no cavities and are somewhat moveable.	growth zones in the arms and legs

synovial joints	Have joint cavities that are kept lubricated by synovial fluid.	intercarpal joint
plane joints	Joints that glide where the flat ends of bones connect.	intertarsal joints
uniaxial joints	Allow movement around one axis only.	elbow joint
biaxial joints	Allow movement around two axes.	knee joint
multiaxial joints	Allow movement around three axes.	ball-and-socket joint found in the hip and shoulder

A joint is an area where two or more bones come together. This contact point creates an important relationship with respect to the body's ability to move. If any of the bones in a joint do not function properly, the joint will not be able to operate as a unit (not all joints, however, are made for movement). There are three kinds of joints: fibrous joints (nonmoveable), cartilaginous joints (somewhat moveable), and synovial joints (very moveable).

Fibrous Joints

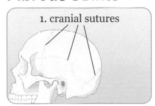
1. cranial sutures

There are two types of fibrous joints: suture and syndesmosis. A fibrous joint has no joint cavity and, in general, does not move. Examples of fibrous joints include cranial sutures and the radioulnar and tibiofibular joints.

Cartilaginous Joints

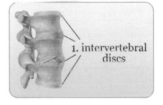
1. intervertebral discs

There are two types of cartilaginous joints: synchondrosis and symphysis. Although a cartilaginous joint has no cavity, it is still somewhat moveable. Examples of cartilaginous joints are the growth zones in the arms and legs, and the disks between the vertebrae.

Synovial Joints

There are four types of synovial joints: plane, uniaxial, biaxial, and multiaxial A synovial joint has a joint cavity that is kept lubricated by synovial fluid. The looser the joint, the more unstable and susceptible it is to injury or other damage. The body compensates for the weakness in synovial joints with ligaments, tendons, and muscle overlays. In this way, joints can be strengthened and supported to a much higher degree, yet still be capable of functioning freely.

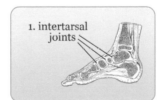
1. intertarsal joints

Plane joints are joints that glide where the flat ends of bones connect. Examples of plane joints are the intercarpal and intertarsal joints.

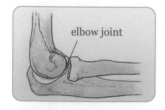

elbow joint

Uniaxial joints allow movement around one axis only. Examples of uniaxial joints are the elbow joint and the interphalangeal joint.

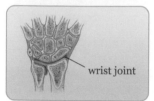

wrist joint

Biaxial joints allow movement around two axes. Examples of biaxial joints are the knee joint, the temporomandibular (jaw) joint, and the radiocarpal (wrist) joint.

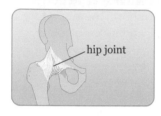

hip joint

Multiaxial joints allow movement around three axes. Examples of multiaxial joints are the ball and socket joint found in the hip and shoulder, as well as the carpometacarpal joint of the thumb between the trapezium (base of thumb) and the first metacarpal. Ball-and-socket joints are the most freely moveable joints in the body.

I. **TRUE/FALSE.**
   Mark the following true or false.

1. A biaxial joint is a type of synovial joint
   ○ true
   ○ false

2. Fibrous joints do not move.
   ○ true
   ○ false

3. Synovial joints have no cavities and are somewhat moveable.
   ○ true
   ○ false

4. The elbow is an example of a uniaxial joint.
   ○ true
   ○ false

5. A cranial suture is an example of cartilaginous joints.
   ○ true
   ○ false

II. **FILL IN THE BLANK.**
   Using the word/word parts in the box, fill in the blanks.

| suture and syndesmosis |
| cartilaginous |
| ligaments |
| synovial |
| biaxial |

1. A multiaxial joint has a joint cavity kept lubricated by

   _____ fluid.

2. The two types of fibrous joints are _____.

3. Synchondrosis and symphysis are examples of

   _____ joints.

4. The knee joint is an example of a _____ joint.

5. The body compensates for potential weakness in synovial joints

   with _____ tendons and muscle overlays.

Joint Movement

Along with the many different types of joints in the body, there are many different ways in which joints move. These are often noted in the physical examination of patients with aches, pains, and difficulty with movement.

Take a moment to try each of these joint movements. What are you doing when you pick up a gallon of milk? What about when you reach for an item from a high shelf?

I. **TERMINOLOGY.**
   Enter each term in the space provided. Read the definition and description for each term.

1. **flexion** _____ _____

   Bending to decrease the angle between two bones. Think of this as "flexing" the biceps.

2. **extension** _____

   Unbending to increase the angle between two bones. Think of this as extending, as in reaching your arm as far as you can (virtually eliminating the angle between the humerus and the radius/ulna).

3. **abduction** _____

   Moving a body part away from the midline.

4. **adduction** _____

   Moving a body part toward the midline. (Think of this as adding a body part back to the body.)

5. **circumduction** _____

   Movement of a body part in a circle, which can include all the above joint movements as well.

II. MATCHING.
Match the correct term to the definition.

1. ____ extension
2. ____ flexion
3. ____ abduction
4. ____ adduction
5. ____ circumduction

A. circling
B. bending
C. moving away from midline
D. adding a part back to the body
E. unbending

III. FILL IN THE BLANK.
Use the word(s) in the box to fill in the blanks.

1. Moving your hand into a fist is considered _____.

2. From a sitting position, bring one foot up to the level of the knee. This is _____.

3. A great back stretch would be bending from the waist toward the right, and circling all the way around. This is called

   _____.

4. _____ would be used in raising your arm straight out to the side.

5. Bringing the ankles together from a wide stance is leg

   _____

circumduction
adduction
extension
flexion
abduction

IV. FILL IN THE BLANK.
Enter the bolded terms in the space provided.

1. **rotation** _____ Movement of a body part or parts around its axis (movement from side to side with the lower body stationary).

2. **supine** _____ The position of the body when lying face up, including hands being palm up and feet bent upwards.

3. **prone** _____ The position of the body when lying face down, including the hands being palm down and the feet bent downwards.

66

4. **dorsiflexion** _____ Movement of the foot that brings the top of the foot closer to the leg.

5. **plantar flexion** _____ Movement of the foot that brings the heel closer to the posterior part of the leg, the toe pointed farther away from the leg. This is the opposite of dorsiflexion.

V. MATCHING.
Match the correct term to the definition.

1. ____ dorsiflexion
2. ____ plantar flexion
3. ____ rotation
4. ____ supine
5. ____ prone

A. lying face down
B. lying face up
C. pointing the toe
D. flexing the toe
E. around an axis

VI. FILL IN THE BLANK.
Use the word(s) in the box to fill in the blanks.

1. Lying face down, as necessary for back surgery, is considered

   _____ .

2. _____ is movement around an axis or stationary point.

3. In a chorus line, dancers must always use _____ .

4. In karate, in order to avoid breaking the toes, an athlete must use _____ .

5. Surgery on the chest cavity would require the patient to be placed in _____ .

| plantar flexion |
| flexion |
| supine |
| prone |
| rotation |
| dorsiflexion |

VII. MULTIPLE CHOICE.
Choose the best answer.

1. Dorsiflexion is:
   - ○ Movement of the foot that brings the heel closer to the posterior part of the leg.
   - ○ Movement of a body part in a circle.
   - ○ Movement of a body part on its axis.
   - ○ Movement of the foot that brings the top of the foot closer to the leg.

2. Synovial joints _____.
   - ○ rarely move
   - ○ move with ease
   - ○ never move
   - ○ only move from the hips

3. Bending to decrease the angle between bones is called _____.
   - ○ extension
   - ○ abduction
   - ○ flexion
   - ○ plantar flexion

4. Circumduction is _____.
   - ○ movement on the axis
   - ○ movement in a circle
   - ○ movement towards the midline
   - ○ unbending to increase the angle between two bones

5. The position of the body when lying face down, including the hands being palm down and the feet bent downwards, is called _____.
   - ○ rested
   - ○ prone
   - ○ flat
   - ○ supine

6. An area where two bones move is called a _____.
   - ○ suture
   - ○ joint
   - ○ synovial
   - ○ facet

7. The three types of joints are _____.
   ○ fibrous, fractured, synovial
   ○ synovial, cartilaginous, simple
   ○ fibrous, cartilaginous, synovial
   ○ syndesmosis, cartilaginous, fibrous

8. Plane joints are _____.
   ○ cartilaginous joints
   ○ fibrous joints
   ○ synovial joints
   ○ symphysis joints

9. Joints that allow movement around three axes are called _____.
   ○ uniaxial
   ○ triaxial
   ○ biaxial
   ○ multiaxial

10. Cartilaginous joints are _____.
    ○ freely moveable
    ○ somewhat moveable
    ○ generally not moveable

Articulations

In most joints, the contacting surfaces of the bones are protected with layers of cartilage. Cartilage is a specialized fibrous connective tissue needed for both the development and growth of bones. Some of the terms in this list are made up of one or more types of cartilage. Some of the terms listed below describe junctions of bone with cartilage, as well as the junctions of one piece or type of cartilage with another.

The following is a list of common articulations. These are terms you may frequently read in reports, and each is followed by the word "joint" or "junction." This is by no means a complete list.

acromioclavicular	glenohumeral	metacarpophalangeal
atlantoaxial	humeroradial	patellofemoral
calcaneocuboid	humeroulnar	radiocarpal
carpometacarpal	iliofemoral	radioulnar
costochondral	iliosacral	sacroiliac
costovertebral	incudomalleolar	sternoclavicular
cricoarytenoid	incudostapedial	talonavicular
cricothyroid	intercarpal	tarsometatarsal
cubitoradial	interphalangeal	temporomandibular
cuneocuboid	manubriosternal	tibiofibular
cuneonavicular		

You will undoubtedly have recognized parts of familiar terms in this list. You should already be able to see your study of medical terminology coming in handy.

I. FILL IN THE BLANK.
Enter the bolded terms in the space provided.

1. **acromioclavicular** _____
2. **atlantoaxial** _____
3. **calcaneocuboid** _____
4. **carpometacarpal** _____
5. **costochondral** _____
6. **costovertebral** _____
7. **cricoarytenoid** _____
8. **cricothyroid** _____
9. **cubitoradial** _____
10. **cuneocuboid** _____
11. **cuneonavicular** _____
12. **glenohumeral** _____
13. **humeroradial** _____
14. **humeroulnar** _____
15. **iliofemoral** _____
16. **iliosacral** _____
17. **incudomalleolar** _____
18. **incudostapedial** _____
19. **intercarpal** _____
20. **interphalangeal** _____
21. **manubriosternal** _____
22. **metacarpophalangeal** _____
23. **patellofemoral** _____
24. **radiocarpal** _____
25. **radioulnar** _____
26. **sacroiliac** _____
27. **sternoclavicular** _____
28. **talonavicular** _____
29. **tarsometatarsal** _____
30. **temporomandibular** _____
31. **tibiofibular** _____

Ligaments

The ligaments are closely related to the skeletal system and are vital to the function of it. They are specifically associated with joints. A ligament is a band of white, fibrous, slightly elastic tissue that binds the ends of bones together. This binding prevents dislocations and stress that can cause fractures.

The word *ligament* comes from the Latin word *ligamentum* meaning to band or tie. A ligament made up of many fibrous bands is called a collateral ligament.

Most ligaments derive their names from the area where they are located, their shape, or the bones and/or structures near that area. For example, there is a carpal ligament in the wrist and a series of cervical ligaments in the neck, which are terms that, by now, should be somewhat familiar to you.

Because of the repetition that occurs in the naming of individual ligaments, there is no reason to map out and memorize each and every individual ligament in the body. Instead, we will deal specifically with two types of ligaments:

1. those that are susceptible to injury
2. ligaments that are studied in common injuries and the terms that are related to them.

There are many ligaments that are not listed here. As you become more familiar with human anatomy, most of the ligaments will become familiar to you as well. You will be able to recognize the names as similar to the names of surrounding structures, shapes, and positions (such as anterior or lateral).

I. TERMINOLOGY.
Enter each term in the space provided. Read the definition and description for each term.

1. **accessory ligament** _____

Any ligament that strengthens or supports another ligament.

2. **arcuate ligament** _____

Means curved or bow-shaped ligaments; they are located in the spine and assist in maintaining the erect position. (Also called ligamenta flava [plural], and ligamentum flavum [singular].)

3. **collateral ligament** _____

There are several types of collateral ligaments, including fibular, radial, tibial, ulnar, etc. These are basically ligaments that are not direct, but are supporting ligaments.

4. **coracoid ligament** _____

Coracoid means like a raven's beak and is used to describe an area on the scapula. It is so named for its shape.

5. **cruciate ligament** _____

Cruciate means shaped like a cross. There are different types of cruciate ligaments, including anterior, posterior, and lateral. They appear in many places in human anatomy, such as the knees, fingers, and toes.

6. **falciform ligament** _____

Falciform means shaped like a sickle and appears near the sacral tuberosity as well as within the liver.

7. **inguinal ligament** _____

Inguinal is a term used to describe the groin area.

8. **interosseous ligament** _____

Interosseous means between bones and describes several different ligaments.

9. **longitudinal ligament** _____

Longitudinal simply means lengthwise. It is used to describe any ligament that runs lengthwise.

10. **nuchal ligament** _____

Nuchal means pertaining to the neck.

11. **triquetral ligament** _____

Triquetral means three cornered and appears in different places throughout the body. The prefix tri- should be familiar as meaning three.

II. MATCHING.
Match the correct term to the definition.

1. ____ cruciate
2. ____ arcuate
3. ____ accessory
4. ____ coracoid
5. ____ collateral

A. shaped like a cross
B. support
C. indirect
D. like a raven's beak
E. curved or bow-shaped ligament

III. FILL IN THE BLANK.
Use the word(s) in the box to fill in the blanks.

1. An area of the scapula is shaped like a bird's beak. The ligament that surrounds it is called the _____ ligament.

2. An _____ ligament strengthens or supports another ligament.

3. A _____ ligament is shaped like a cross.

4. Located on the spine, the _____ ligament literally means "curved or bow-shaped ligament."

5. There are several types of _____ ligaments that are made up of several bands and are not directly connected.

| accessory |
| collateral |
| cruciate |
| coracoid |
| arcuate |

IV. MATCHING.

1. ____ falciform
2. ____ nuchal
3. ____ interosseous
4. ____ triquetral
5. ____ inguinal
6. ____ longitudinal

A. the neck
B. lengthwise
C. sickle-shaped
D. groin area
E. three cornered
F. between bones

V. FILL IN THE BLANK.
Use the word(s) in the box to fill in the blanks.

1. If a ligament runs along the length of a bone, it is usually called
   a _____ ligament.

2. Within the liver, the _____ ligament is shaped like
   a sickle.

3. Many ligaments, by virtue of their function to support and
   strengthen the skeletal system, run in between bones. These are
   called _____ ligaments.

4. A _____ ligament is found in the neck.

5. Three-cornered or _____ ligaments are found
   throughout the body.

6. The _____ ligament is found in the groin area.

falciform
triquetral
longitudinal
inguinal
nuchal
interosseous

Fractures – Lesson 1

The skeletal system is susceptible to injury, trauma, and
disease. When we think of bone injuries or problems, the
first thing that comes to mind is probably a fracture. A
fracture is a break or a rupture in a bone. There are many
types of fractures. If you review radiology reports, clinic
notes, or emergency room reports, you will see a wide
variety of different types of fractures, as they occur
frequently.

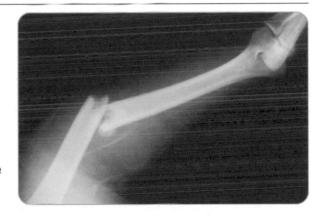

The fractures presented here are by no means a complete
list. There are many other types of fractures that are not
listed here. Some fractures have been delineated by
proper names and are specific to a particular bone. If you
come across a fracture that is completely unfamiliar to you, the best place to look is in a dictionary or word list
under the heading *fracture*. Closely related to fractures are dislocations. While the term *dislocation* refers to a
general displacement of any body part, it is most commonly associated with a bone displacement. Often
displacements are categorized or named with the same names given to fractures.

I. TERMINOLOGY.

Enter the fracture in the space provided, and be sure that you spell it correctly.
The "f" following the term is simply an abbreviation for the word "fracture" and should not be included in your answer.

1. **apophyseal f.** _____

A fracture in which a small fragment is torn from the bone.

2. **articular f.** _____

A fracture of the joint surface.

3. **avulsion f.** _____

An indirect fracture caused by tearing or pulling of a ligament.

4. **blow-out f.** _____

A fracture of the orbital floor caused by traumatic force.

5. **boxer f.** _____

Fracture of the metacarpal neck, caused by striking something hard with a closed fist.

6. **bucket-handle f.** _____

Also called a "bucket-handle tear," it is a tear in the cartilage and it leaves a loop of cartilage lying in the intercondylar notch.

7. **burst f.** _____

Also called an "axial compression fracture," it is a fracture of a vertebra, often injuring the spinal cord.

8. **butterfly f.** _____

A comminuted fracture resulting in two fragments of bone on either side of a main fragment; the result resembles a butterfly.

II. SPELLING.

Determine if the following words are spelled correctly. If the spelling is correct, leave the word as it has already been entered. If the spelling is incorrect, provide the correct spelling.

1. fragment _____   2. fracter _____

3. blow-out _____   4. butterfly _____

5. articuler _____

III. MULTIPLE CHOICE.
Choose the best answer.

1. A fracture of the joint surface is an (◯articular, ◯avulsion) fracture.

2. A butterfly fracture is a (◯comminuted, ◯communicated) fracture resulting in two fragments of bone on either side of a main fragment.

3. A burst fracture is also referred to as a/an (◯skeletal, ◯axial) compression fracture.

4. A fracture in which a small fragment is torn from the bone is an (◯apophysial, ◯ apophyseal) fracture.

5. An avulsion fracture is a/an (◯direct, ◯indirect) fracture.

Fractures – Lesson 2

I. TERMINOLOGY.
Enter the fracture in the space provided, and be sure that you spell it correctly.
The "f" following the term is simply an abbreviation for the word "fracture" and should not be included in your answer.

1. **buttonhole f.** _____
Also called a "perforating fracture," it results when a bone is perforated by a missile.

2. **chisel f.** _____
Detachment of a piece from the head of the radius.

3. **cleavage f.** _____
Shelling off of cartilage by a small fragment of bone.

4. **closed f.** _____
A fracture that does not penetrate or produce an open wound in the skin.

5. **Colles' f.** _____
Fracture of the lower end of the radius, where the fragment is displaced.

6. **comminuted f.** _____
A fracture in which the bone is splintered or crushed.

7. **complete f.** _____
A fracture in which the bone is entirely broken all the way across.

8. **complicated f.** _____
When there is injury to adjacent parts of the bone due to a fracture.

II. SPELLING.
Determine if the following words are spelled correctly. If the spelling is correct, leave the word as it has already been entered. If the spelling is incorrect, provide the correct spelling.

1. button hole _____

2. cleevage _____

3. closed _____

4. complecated _____

5. colles _____

III. MATCHING.
Match the correct term to the definition.

1. ____ Also called a perforating fracture.

2. ____ A fracture in which the bone is splintered or crushed.

3. ____ A fracture in which the bone is completely broken, all the way across.

4. ____ Fracture of the lower end of the radius with displaced fragment.

5. ____ Detached piece of bone from the head of the radius.

A. complete
B. buttonhole
C. chisel
D. Colles'
E. comminuted

Fractures – Lesson 3

I. TERMINOLOGY.
Enter the fracture in the space provided, and be sure that you spell it correctly.
The "f" following the term is simply an abbreviation for the word "fracture" and should not be included in your answer.

1. **compound f.** _____
Basically just an open fracture.

2. **compression f.** _____
A fracture as a result of compression.

3. **condylar f.** _____
A fracture of the humerus where a small fragment that includes the condyle is separated from the bone.

4. **dislocation f.** _____
A fracture that occurs near a joint and results in displacement of the joint.

5. **greenstick f.** _____

Also called "hickory-stick fracture," it is a fracture in which one side of the bone is broken and the other side is bent.

6. **hangman's f.** _____

A fracture through the axis (C2).

7. **impacted f.** _____

When one fragment of a fracture is driven into another.

8. **indirect f.** _____

A fracture that occurs at a point distant from the injury.

II. **SPELLING.**
   Determine if the following words are spelled correctly. If the spelling is correct, leave the word as it has already been entered. If the spelling is incorrect, provide the correct spelling.

1. condalyr _____   2. disslocation _____

3. hangmen's _____   4. greensteck _____

5. axis _____

III. **TRUE/FALSE.**
   Mark the following true or false.

   1. A fracture that occurs at a point distant from the injury is called a direct fracture.
      ◯ true
      ◯ false

   2. A compression fracture is a fracture as a result of a compression
      ◯ true
      ◯ false

   3. A greenstick fracture Is also referred to an oak-stick fracture.
      ◯ true
      ◯ false

4. When one fragment of a fracture is driven into another this is an impacted fracture.
    ○ true
    ○ false

5. An open fracture is generally referred to as a compound fracture.
    ○ true
    ○ false

Fractures – Lesson 4

I. **TERMINOLOGY.**
    Enter the fracture in the space provided, and be sure that you spell it correctly.
    The "f" following the term is simply an abbreviation for the word "fracture" and should not be included in your answer.

    1. **insufficiency f.** _____

    A stress fracture that occurs when there is a normal amount of stress, but the bone is of decreased density.

    2. **intra-articular f.** _____

    A fracture on the articular surface of a bone (also acceptably presented as intraarticular).

    3. **intracapsular f.** _____

    A fracture occurring within the capsule of a joint.

    4. **intrauterine f.** _____

    Fracture of a fetal bone while in utero.

    5. **Le Fort f.** _____

    Fracture of the maxilla. (There are different types of Le Fort fractures; they are dictated "Le Fort 1, 2, or 3" and are transcribed as Le Fort I, Le Fort II, and Le Fort III.)

    6. **linear f.** _____

    A fracture extending along the length of a bone.

    7. **longitudinal f.** _____

    A break extending in a longitudinal direction.

    8. **oblique f.** _____

    A break extending in an oblique direction.

II. TRUE/FALSE.
The following terms are spelled correctly: true or false?

1. insufficiency
   - ○ true
   - ○ false

2. Lefort
   - ○ true
   - ○ false

3. lineare
   - ○ true
   - ○ false

4. oblicque
   - ○ true
   - ○ false

5. longitudinal
   - ○ true
   - ○ false

III. FILL IN THE BLANK.
Using the word(s) in the box, enter the appropriate term in the space provided.

1. An intrauterine fracture occurs in _____.

2. The _____ of a joint is affected in an intracapsular fracture.

3. A fracture on the articular surface of a bone is classified as _____.

4. An insufficiency fracture which occurs when the bone is of decreased _____.

5. A Le Fort fracture involves the _____.

capsule
density
intra-articular
maxilla
utero

Fractures – Lesson 5

I. **TERMINOLOGY.**
   Enter the fracture in the space provided, and be sure that you spell it correctly.
   The "f" following the term is simply an abbreviation for the word "fracture" and should not be included in your answer.

1. **open f.** _____
   A fracture that results in an external wound (i.e., a portion of the fractured bone protrudes through the skin).

2. **simple f.** _____
   Opposite of a compound fracture; basically a closed fracture.

3. **spiral f.** _____
   Also called a "torsion fracture," it is where a bone is literally twisted apart.

4. **spontaneous f.** _____
   Occurs as a result of some longstanding disease and is not traumatic.

5. **stress f.** _____
   Caused as a result of repeated stress to a bone (commonly seen in soldiers or athletes).

6. **subcapital f.** _____
   A fracture of a bone just below its head.

7. **torsion f.** _____
   Also called a "spiral fracture." See above.

8. **torus f.** _____
   A fracture with localized expansion of the cortex, but little or no displacement of the lower end of the bone.

9. **transverse f.** _____
   A fracture that occurs at a right angle to the axis of a bone.

10. **tuft f.** _____
    A splintered fracture of the distal phalanx.

II. SPELLING.
Determine if the following words are spelled correctly. If the spelling is correct, leave the word as it has already been entered. If the spelling is incorrect, provide the correct spelling.

1. stress _____

2. spirel _____

3. open _____

4. toris _____

5. tramatic _____

III. MULTIPLE CHOICE.
Choose the best answer.

1. Another term for a spiral fracture.
   - ○ torshun
   - ○ torsoin
   - ○ torsion
   - ○ torsioun

2. A fracture just below the head of a bone.
   - ○ subcappital
   - ○ subcapital
   - ○ subcapitle
   - ○ subcappille

3. Fracture resulting from a longstanding disease (not traumatic).
   - ○ spontanious
   - ○ spontaneus
   - ○ sponteanus
   - ○ spontancous

4. A fracture that occurs at the right angle to the axis of a bone.
   - ○ transverse
   - ○ transferse
   - ○ transversal
   - ○ transference

5. A splintered fracture of the distal phalanx.
   - ○ tuff
   - ○ tuf
   - ○ tuft
   - ○ tift

Musculoskeletal Diseases – Lesson 1

Obviously, there are other problems besides fractures and dislocations that can afflict the skeletal system. Following is a list of some of these disease processes. These maladies can be seen most often in orthopedics, neurology, internal medicine, pediatrics, hematology/oncology, and geriatrics. However, the terms may appear in virtually any other specialty as well.

I. TERMINOLOGY.
   Enter each term in the space provided. Read the definition and description for each term.

   1. **achondroplasia** _____

   A hereditary disorder of cartilage and bone formation.
   Symptoms are disproportionately short limbs.

   2. **ankylosing spondylitis** _____

   This is a rheumatoid arthritis of the spine. It is progressive and is found most often in young men, affecting the intervertebral joints, the sacroiliac joints, and the costovertebral joints.
   Symptoms are back pain and early morning stiffness relieved by activity.

   3. **arthritis** _____

   This affects joints and is the inflammation of one or more joints. There are many types. The most common is osteoarthritis.
   Symptoms include joint pain, swelling, stiffness, deformity, fever, and weight loss.

   4. **inflammation** _____

   A response of body tissues to injury or irritation; characterized by pain, swelling, redness and heat.

   5. **rheumatoid** _____

   A type of arthritis characterized by inflammatory changes throughout the body's connective tissues.

   6. **chondrosarcoma** _____

   This is a malignant tumor of cartilage.
   Symptoms include pain and generally the presence of a mass.

   7. **degenerative joint disease** _____

   Joint disease characterized by degeneration of the articular cartilage.
   Symptoms include pain and stiffness in joints which is aggravated with physical activity and relieved with rest.

   8. **Ewing tumor** _____

   This is a cancerous tumor or malignancy that invades the entire shaft of the bone.
   Symptoms include pain and swelling.

   9. **sarcoma** _____

   A connective tissue tumor that is usually malignant.

II. SPELLING.

Determine if the following words are spelled correctly. If the spelling is correct, leave the word as it has already been entered. If the spelling is incorrect, provide the correct spelling.

1. achondraplasia _____   2. rhuematoid _____

3. degeneretive _____   4. inflammation _____

5. Ewwing _____

III. MULTIPLE CHOICE.

Choose the best answer.

1. A Ewing tumor is a (◯noncancerous, ◯cancerous) tumor that invades the entire shaft of the bone.

2. The most common type of arthritis is (◯osteoarthritis, ◯chondrosarcoma).

3. Degenerative joint disease is characterized by degeneration of the (◯articular, ◯ epiphyseal) cartilage.

4. Rheumatoid arthritis of the spine is referred to as (◯ankylosing, ◯anklyosing) spondylitis.

5. Arthritis is inflammation of one or more (◯bones, ◯joints).

Musculoskeletal Diseases – Lesson 2

I. TERMINOLOGY.

Enter the term in the space provided, and be sure that you spell it correctly.

1. **gout** _____

A systemic disease due to deposition of urate crystals.
Symptoms include episodes of severe pain and swelling, usually affecting a single joint.

2. **Hurler syndrome** _____

This is caused by irregular ossification and is due to an overproduction of mucopolysaccharides.
Symptoms include short stature, coarse features, skeletal deformities, enlarged organs.

3. **mucopolysaccharides** _____

An antiarthritic compound that effectively increases the viscosity (or stickiness) of synovial fluid.

4. **hypophosphatasia** _____

This condition is a result of a deficiency in alkaline phosphatase.
Symptoms include skeletal defects, bone pain, and other abnormal body chemistries.

5. **alkaline phosphatase** _____

Enzyme produced in the bone and liver.

6. **Legg-Calve-Perthes disease** _____

Disease of the hip joint that results in a loss of bone mass due to inadequate blood flow to the joint. *Symptoms include hip or groin pain which is aggravated with physical activity. A limp is often the result of the severe pain.*

7. **Marfan syndrome** _____

This results from abnormal formation of connective tissue.
Symptoms include long, slender habitus, skeletal malformations, and vision/eye problems.

II. **SPELLING.**
Determine if the following words are spelled correctly. If the spelling is correct, leave the word as it has already been entered. If the spelling is incorrect, provide the correct spelling.

1. guot _____   2. mucopolysacharides _____

3. alkaline phosphatase _____   4. hurler _____

5. systemec _____

III. **MATCHING.**
Match the term to the appropriate symptoms.

1. ____ Severe pain and swelling, usually affecting a single joint.

2. ____ Skeletal defects, bone pain and other abnormal body chemistries.

3. ____ Hip pain and limping.

4. ____ Short stature, coarse features, skeletal deformities, enlarged organs.

5. ____ Long slender habitus, skeletal malformations, and vision/eye problems.

A. Hurler syndrome
B. hypophosphatasia
C. Marfan syndrome
D. gout
E. Legg-Calve-Perthes disease

Musculoskeletal Diseases – Lesson 3

I. TERMINOLOGY.
Enter the term in the space provided, and be sure that you spell it correctly.

1. **multiple myeloma** _____

This is the most common bone neoplasm. It is a tumor derived from the blood cells.
Symptoms include pain and swelling.

2. **Osgood-Schlatter disease** _____

This disease affects the tibial tubercle, where the patella inserts onto the tibia. It manifests itself when growth centers become stressed (usually due to physical/athletic activity).
Symptoms include limping and pain at the site upon exertion.

3. **osteochondritis dissecans** _____

This is the term for osteochondrosis (see below) involving the joints, particularly the shoulder and knee joints.

4. **osteochondrosis** _____

This is a general term for a group of developmental disorders that affect ossification centers and usually occur in adolescence. Some of these include Legg-Calve-Perthes disease, Osgood-Schlatter disease, and Scheuermann disease.
Major symptoms include pain and limited movement of the affected joints or bones.

5. **osteogenesis imperfecta** _____

This is also a result of abnormal formation of connective tissues.
Symptoms include blue sclerae, fractures as a result of very minor trauma, and deafness.

6. **osteoid osteoma** _____

This is a benign lesion that can occur in any bone, but is most common in the long bones.
Symptoms include skeletal deformities, bowing of long bones, and hypertrophy of epiphyses.

7. **osteomalacia** _____

This is softening of bone as a result of the bone being poorly mineralized.
Symptoms include deformities and fractures of bones.

8. **osteomyelitis** _____

This is usually a bacterial infection of the bone, although it can also be a fungal infection. The most common pathogen is the bacteria Staphylococcus aureus.
Symptoms include the onset of bone pain, fever, and chills. (Incidentally, most infections are recognizable by the presence of fever and chills.)

9. **Staphylococcus aureus** _____

Bacteria of the genus Staphylococcus, it is found in nasal membranes, skin, hair follicles, and perineum.

II. SPELLING.

Determine if the following words are spelled correctly. If the spelling is correct, leave the word as it has already been entered. If the spelling is incorrect, provide the correct spelling.

1. Osgood-Sclatter _____

2. osteochrondrosis _____

3. osteochrondritis _____

4. Staphylococus _____

5. neoplasm _____

III. MULTIPLE CHOICE.

Choose the best answer.

1. Abnormal formation of connective tissue.

   ○ osteogenesis imprefecta
   ○ ostiogenesis imprefecta
   ○ osteogenesis imperfecta
   ○ ostiogenesis imperfecta

2. The most common bone neoplasm.

   ○ multiple myeloma
   ○ multiple meyloma
   ○ multiple myleoma
   ○ multiple myloma

3. Usually a bacterial infection of the bone, although it can also be a fungal infection.

   ○ osteomielitis
   ○ osteomyelitis
   ○ osteomylitis
   ○ osteomyleitis

4. A benign lesion which can occur in any bone.

   ○ osteoid osteoma
   ○ osteod osteoma
   ○ ostioud osteoma
   ○ osteoid ostemoa

5. A softening of bone.

   ○ osteomalcia
   ○ osteomalcea
   ○ osteomalacea
   ○ osteomalacia

Musculoskeletal Diseases – Lesson 4

I. **TERMINOLOGY.**
   Enter the term in the space provided, and be sure that you spell it correctly.

1. **osteoporosis** _____

This occurs when the density of the bone is inadequate to allow for the proper support required of bone.
Symptoms include backache, loss of height, and forward hunching of the spine (which is called kyphosis).

2. **kyphosis** _____

Forward hunching of the spine.

3. **Paget disease** _____

A degenerative disorder of the bone resulting in the softening and swelling of bone.
Symptoms include bone pain, kyphosis, bowing of the shins, and cranial swelling. (The cranial swelling specifically can lead to deafness.)

4. **psoriatic arthritis** _____

Psoriasis is a chronic skin disease which causes scaling, dryness, pustules, and abscesses to appear on the nails, scalp, lumbar area of the spine, and genitalia. This can lead to joint involvement, which is psoriatic arthritis.

5. **Reiter syndrome** _____

This is an arthritis associated with nonbacterial urethritis, conjunctivitis, cervicitis, and mucocutaneous lesions. It is pronounced "writer" syndrome, but should never be spelled this way.
Symptoms are different depending upon the etiology of the syndrome, particularly whether it arises first as a urethritis or cervicitis (in the reproductive system); conjunctivitis is the most common lesion of the eye, and mucocutaneous lesions are superficial ulcers.

6. **rickets** _____

Occurs in infants as a result of overgrowth of poorly mineralized bone and enlarged marrow cavities.
Symptoms include skeletal deformities, bowing of long bones, and hypertrophy of epiphyses.

7. **Scheuermann disease** _____

This disease specifically affects the ossification centers of the vertebrae.
Symptoms include juvenile kyphosis, or a curved appearance of the spine.

8. **scoliosis** _____

Scoliosis is lateral (or sideways) curvature of the spine in the erect position. It is caused by malalignment of the vertebrae.

II. **SPELLING.**
Determine if the following words are spelled correctly. If the spelling is correct, leave the word as it has already been entered. If the spelling is incorrect, provide the correct spelling.

1. paget _____   2. rackets _____

3. psoriatic _____   4. Scheurmann _____

5. artheritis _____

III. **MATCHING.**
Match the correct term to the definition.

1. ____ Forward hunching of the spine.

2. ____ Overgrowth of poorly mineralized bone and enlarged marrow cavities in infants.

3. ____ Affects the ossification centers of the vertebrae.

4. ____ Occurs when density of bone is inadequate to allow for proper support.

5. ____ Lateral curvature of the spine in the erect position.

A. Scheuermann disease
B. rickets
C. scoliosis
D. kyphosis
E. osteoporosis

Review: Musculoskeletal Diseases

I. **MULTIPLE CHOICE.**
Choose the best answer.

1. An arthritis associated with nonbacterial urethritis, conjunctivitis, cervicitis, and mucocutaneous lesions.
   ○ Scheuermann disease
   ○ Osgood-Schlatter disease
   ○ Reiter syndrome
   ○ osteochondrosis

2. Lateral curvature of the spine in the erect position caused by malalignment of the vertebrae.
   ○ rickets
   ○ scoliosis
   ○ kyphosis
   ○ osteomalacia

3. A systemic disease due to deposition of urate crystals. Symptoms include episodes of severe pain and swelling, usually affecting a single joint.
   - ○ hypophosphatasia
   - ○ gout
   - ○ Legg-Calve-Perthes disease
   - ○ psoriatic arthritis

4. A degenerate disorder of the bone resulting in the softening and swelling of bone.
   - ○ Paget disease
   - ○ Reiter syndrome
   - ○ Ewing tumor
   - ○ Hurler syndrome

5. A hereditary disorder of cartilage and bone formation causing disproportionately short limbs.
   - ○ sarcoma
   - ○ Marfan syndrome
   - ○ achondroplasia
   - ○ osteochondrosis

II. MATCHING.
Match the correct term to the definition.

1. ____ a malignant tumor of cartilage

2. ____ condition that is a result of deficiency in alkaline phosphatase

3. ____ forward hunching of the spine

4. ____ bacterial infection of the bone; can also be a fungal infection

5. ____ occurs in infants as a result of overgrowth of poorly mineralized bone and enlarged marrow cavities

6. ____ a benign lesion that can occur in any bone, but is most common in the long bones

7. ____ affects joints and is the inflammation of one or more joints

8. ____ joint disease characterized by degeneration of the articular cartilage

A. rickets
B. chondrosarcoma
C. degenerative joint disease
D. hypophosphatasia
E. kyphosis
F. arthritis
G. osteoid osteoma
H. osteomyelitis

III. SPELLING.

Determine if the following words are spelled correctly. If the spelling is correct, leave the word as it has already been entered. If the spelling is incorrect, retype the word with the correct spelling.

1. Uing tumor _____

2. Leg-Calf-Perths disease _____

3. ostiogenesis imperficta _____

4. kifosis _____

5. Writer syndrome _____

6. sculiosis _____

7. rumatoid _____

8. soriatic arthritis _____

Unit 4
Muscular System

Muscular System – Introduction

The skeletal system gives the body the framework for movement and mobility, but the muscles provide the power. A muscle is an organ that contracts to produce movement. Muscle contraction in conjunction with skeletal flexibility makes movement possible in human beings. Without muscles there would be no voluntary movement of the body whatsoever and many internal systems and organs would be unable to function.

Let's take a look at the organs of the body that provide the power.

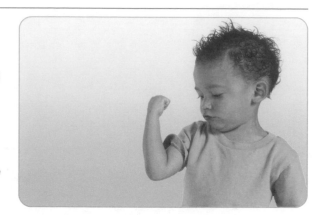

Function and Types

Muscle tissue has the following functions:

- **Movement**. Muscles that attach to the human skeleton allow us to walk, run, jump, and otherwise voluntarily move about. Muscles that form the walls of many visceral organs produce movement by involuntarily contracting and relaxing, thereby squeezing body fluids and other substances through various organs (e.g., the esophagus, stomach, intestines, blood vessels, etc.).
- **Posture**. In order for the body to maintain an erect posture or a sitting position, certain muscles must contract or remain contracted.
- **Stabilization of joints**. As discussed briefly in the skeletal system, muscles and ligaments are vital to joint stabilization and allow for smooth movement when bending or twisting.
- **Body temperature maintenance**. When muscles contract, they produce heat. Even when the body is at rest, muscles are constantly contracting and producing heat which plays a role in maintaining a normal body temperature of 98.6 degrees Fahrenheit.

There are three different types of muscle tissue found throughout the human body:

- **Skeletal muscle**. The primary muscle used to allow voluntary movement of the body; they are usually attached to the skeleton by tendons.
- **Smooth muscle**. The muscle that lines the walls of internal organs. This muscle is usually short in its strands and allows for the movement of body fluids and waste through the internal systems.
- **Cardiac muscle**. This type of muscle is found only in the heart.

Muscles receive their instructions (stimuli) for movement from the nerves. The nerves contain motor fibers that transmit the impulses from the brain, spinal cord, and sensory fibers for proprioception (perception of the stimuli) to the muscles and connecting tissues. This is the case for both voluntary and involuntary muscle contraction.

I. MATCHING.
Match the correct muscle functions and types to the definition.

1. ___ movement
2. ___ posture
3. ___ stabilization of joints
4. ___ body temperature maintenance
5. ___ skeletal muscle
6. ___ smooth muscle
7. ___ cardiac muscle

A. Muscle found only in the heart
B. When muscles contract and produce heat
C. Primary muscles allowing voluntary movement of the body
D. Allow human skeleton movement
E. Allow for smooth movement when bending or twisting joints
F. Maintain a sitting position
G. Muscles lining the walls of internal organs

Skeletal Muscle

Skeletal muscles are voluntary muscles that connect to the bones of the skeleton. They are termed voluntary because in a normal functioning body, skeletal muscles move when we direct them to move. The cells of skeletal muscle tissue are usually large and have more than one nucleus. Because of their length and thin appearance, these muscle cells are often referred to as fibers (and not cells). Skeletal muscles come in varying shapes and sizes and are called "striated" because of their striped (or band-like) appearance. Although cardiac muscle also appears striped, striated is normally a synonym for voluntary skeletal muscle.

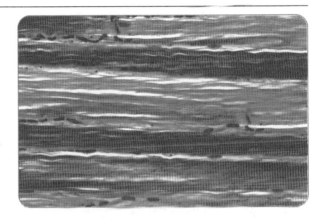

Highlights

The less moveable attachment of a muscle is called the origin. The more moveable attachment of a muscle is called the insertion.

Each muscle is made up of muscle fibers, blood vessels, connective tissue, and nerves. Skeletal muscle fibers are long and thin, often resembling a bunch of sticks that have been grouped together. Each muscle is supplied by at least one nerve, one artery, and (one or more) vein near the center or middle of the muscle.

Most skeletal muscles extend from one bone to another, crossing over at least one joint. When a skeletal muscle crosses a joint and contracts, one bone moves and the other bone remains stationary. The less moveable attachment of a muscle is called the origin. The more moveable attachment of a muscle is called the insertion. The insertion is always pulled towards the origin.

Muscles attach to their origins or insertions via connective tissue that is strong and fibrous. There are two basic types of attachments: direct (fleshy) attachments and indirect attachments. Direct attachments have such short strands of connective tissue that muscles appear to be directly connected to the bone. Indirect attachments are the opposite, with long strands of connective tissue extending far beyond the muscle. These long strands form either a rope-like structure called a tendon, or a flat tissue sheet called an aponeurosis, which connects to the bone. Bones generally have raised markings (tubercles, trochanters, crests) to which tendons attach. Most muscles attach by tendons rather than aponeuroses.

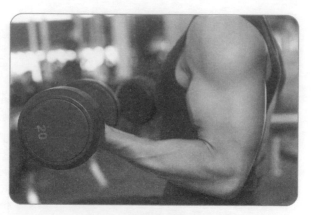

Skeletal muscles are under our direct control. We decide if we want to move an arm or leg, tap our fingers on the table, run, bend, lift, or walk somewhere. Skeletal muscles contract and relax very quickly and are subject to fatigue, depending upon how often or how long they are in use.

Highlights

Bone markings such as tubercles, trochanters, and crests are the places on bone where muscles attach with rope-like tendons. Less commonly, muscles attach with a flat tissue sheet called an aponeurosis.

I. TERMINOLOGY.

Enter each term in the space provided. Read the definition and description for each term.

1. **origin** _____

The less movable attachment of a muscle.

2. **insertion** _____

The more movable attachment of a muscle.

3. **direct (fleshy) attachments** _____

Short strands of connective tissue that make muscles appear as if they are directly connected to the bone.

4. **indirect attachments** _____

Long strands of connective tissue extending beyond the muscle.

5. **tendon** _____

A rope-like structure that binds muscles to bone.

6. **aponeurosis** _____

A flat tissue sheet that connects muscle to bone.

Smooth Muscle

Smooth muscles are found in the internal organs and inside blood vessels. Smooth muscles are involuntary: they contract with stimuli from the nervous system, but without conscious thought. Spindle-like (i.e., length greater than width) and fragile in appearance, smooth muscle cells have a single nucleus. Smooth muscle tissue has no striations. Functions such as blood flow, digestion, and pupillary response are due to smooth muscle contractions.

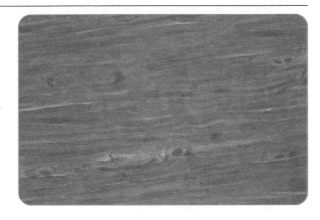

Smooth muscle occupies six major location sites:

- walls of the circulatory vessels
- digestive tubes
- urinary organs
- reproductive organs
- respiratory tubes
- inside the eye

In the hollow visceral organs (such as the digestive tubes), muscle fibers are often grouped into two sheets of smooth muscle. The muscle fibers of the longitudinal layer run parallel to the length of the organ. The muscles of the circular layer wrap around the circumference of the organ. During contraction, the longitudinal layer contracts or shortens the length of the organ, and the circular layer contracts or constricts the hollow organ. These waves of contraction and relaxation cause substances (in the case of the digestive tubes, food, and liquids) to be propelled through these tubes. This process of propelling substances through hollow visceral organs is called peristalsis.

Smooth muscle contraction is slow, sustained, and very resistant to fatigue. Smooth muscle has a slower contraction rate (about 30 times longer than skeletal muscle) but is required to hold such contractions much longer than skeletal muscle. This is important because in many of the internal organs mentioned above, smooth muscle needs to maintain a constant level of contraction.

I. **MULTIPLE CHOICE.**
   Choose the best answer.

1. Smooth muscles are very _____.
   - ◯ easily tired
   - ◯ weak
   - ◯ resistant to fatigue
   - ◯ wide

2. Smooth muscle tissue has no _____.
   - ◯ strength
   - ◯ fibers
   - ◯ tubes
   - ◯ striations

3. Other than in circulatory vessels, smooth muscles can be found in _____.
   ○ the legs
   ○ the eye
   ○ the brain
   ○ the back

4. The process of propelling substances through hollow visceral organs is called _____.
   ○ peristalsis
   ○ hyperstalsis
   ○ contraction
   ○ expansion

5. Smooth muscles are spindle-like, which means they have _____.
   ○ spindled fibers
   ○ faster contractions
   ○ greater width than length
   ○ greater length than width

Cardiac Muscle

Cardiac muscle is the third type of muscle found in the human body and forms the majority of the walls of the heart. It is similar in appearance to skeletal muscle with respect to its striated appearance, but it has a single-cell nucleus. This is an involuntary muscle and direct stimuli from the central nervous system (CNS) is not required for contraction. However, the CNS does modify (not initiate) contraction of cardiac muscle.

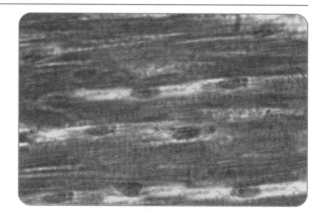

Naming Muscles

The names of muscles are descriptive. Therefore, it will help you to learn and remember them if you have an understanding of how they are named. There are seven (7) primary ways the names assigned to muscles are derived.

Term	Definition	Examples
Shape	Muscle names are often derived from the actual physical shape of the muscle itself or a defining physical characteristic, such as the number of heads that it has.	**Rhomboideus:** A muscle of the back that is shaped like a rhomboid. **Triangularis:** A muscle of the face that is triangular in shape. **Triceps:** A muscle with three (tri-) heads. **Biceps:** A muscle with two (bi-) heads.
Location	A muscle may be named for its actual location within the body relative to other body structures.	**Pectoralis:** Chest muscle located within the pectoral girdle. **Intercostal:** Muscle located between ribs (intercostal literally means between ribs). **Abdominis:** Located in the abdominal area.
Attachment	Many muscles are named for the bones to which they are attached. The muscle name may combine more than one name when more than one bone is involved.	**Zygomaticus:** Attached to the zygoma (bone of the face). **Sternocleidomastoid:** Attached to the sternum, clavicle, and mastoid process of the skull.
Size	The actual size of the muscle or its relative size to a similar muscle may be used in naming a muscle.	**Maximus or Major:** Both of these terms mean larger or largest. **Minimus or Minor:** Meaning smaller or smallest. **Longus:** Meaning long. **Brevis:** Meaning short.
Orientation of fibers	This is the direction that the individual fibers of a muscle extend.	**Oblique:** In a slanting or inclined direction. **Rectus:** Meaning straight. **Transverse:** Meaning across or placed crosswise.

Relative position	These delineations contain basic directional planes and are used on similar muscles to designate a slightly different orientation. Often a "medial" will have a corresponding "lateral"; likewise, an "internal" will have a corresponding "external."	**Lateral:** Something that is further from the midpoint or to the side. **Medial:** Something closer to the middle or the midline. **Internal:** Situated or occurring within or on the inside. **External:** Situated or occurring on the outside.
Function	Muscles are responsible for movement. However, there are several different types of movements, and muscles are often classified according to the actual movement that they produce.	**Adductor:** Movement to draw toward a medial plane. **Extensor:** General term for a muscle that extends a joint. **Flexor:** General term for a muscle that flexes a joint. **Levator:** A muscle that elevates or lifts an organ or structure.

Many muscles are actually part of the musculoskeletal system (muscles of the skeleton). Part of this system has already been introduced. The muscles and bones of the body are interrelated; in fact, they depend upon each other to carry out their individual functions. There are over 600 skeletal muscles in the human body (most of these are voluntary or striated muscles). The good news is that you do not have to know every single muscle in the body (or even just the voluntary ones), although there are some individual muscles that you should know.

You will be encountering maladies associated with the muscles and their surrounding structures in several different specialties. The physical examination specifically examines the musculoskeletal system and is part of virtually any workup. In addition, most surgeries require incisions through various muscle layers. Muscles and tendons themselves can be strained, pulled, torn, infected, and otherwise damaged and need diagnosis, treatment, and care. In other words, a basic understanding of the muscles of the human body will prove extremely beneficial to you in your career as a medical transcription editor.

I. **MATCHING.**
   Match the muscle to the descriptive term that gives it its name.

1. ____ Biceps
2. ____ Abdominis
3. ____ Zygomaticus
4. ____ Longus
5. ____ Rectus
6. ____ Internal
7. ____ Levator

A. Orientation of fibers
B. Shape
C. Location
D. Attachment
E. Size
F. Function
G. Relative position

Anatomical Position

The human body can be looked at from many angles or viewpoints. Therefore, it is necessary for medical personnel to refer to the human body in a fixed or standard position when referring to specific body areas. Descriptive terms for parts of the body are referenced according to this fixed or "anatomical position." The anatomical position refers to the human body as erect (standing), facing forward with eyes straight ahead, arms at the sides with palms open and facing forward, and feet parallel and flat on the floor.

Note that these relative positions are actually used frequently in medical reports. Not only are they used as descriptive words throughout human anatomy, doctors must use them when describing any findings on a physical exam, within an operative note, or when describing an x-ray (where great detail must be provided). In order to achieve clarity of reference, it is necessary for dictators to use standard directional indicators.

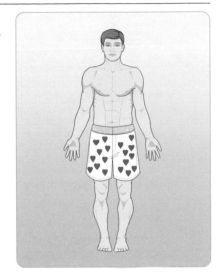

The Anatomical Position

In anatomical terms, any veins, muscles, ligaments, bones, tendons, or other structures that utilize one of these descriptive terms will be specifically related to this anatomical position. If you know and can determine for yourself whether something is above, below, in front of, behind, beside, or near another structure, you can be relatively certain that you are using the correct descriptive term.

I. TERMINOLOGY.
Enter each term in the space provided. Read the definition and description for each term.

1. **anterior** _____

Situated in front of or toward the front of a body part or organ. This term is also used in reference to a ventral or belly surface of the body. Frontal is a common synonym for anterior.

2. **coronal** _____

Division of the body into anterior and posterior sections. Also called frontal plane. Can mean pertaining to the head or the crown.

3. **distal** _____

Remote; farther from any point of reference; opposite of proximal. (The shoulder is distal to the wrist but proximal to the elbow.)

4. **dorsal** _____

Pertaining to the back of the body; also used to denote a position that is more toward the back than another object of reference. Sometimes called posterior.

5. **inferior** _____

Situated below a structure or directed downward; also used to denote the lower portion of an organ or the lower of two structures. Sometimes called caudal.

6. **lateral** _____

Pertaining to the side; denoting a position farther from the midline (median plane) of a structure.

7. **medial** _____

Pertaining to the middle; closer to the midline of a body; pertaining to the middle layer.

8. **posterior** _____

Situated in the back; also used in reference to the back or dorsal surface of the body.

9. **proximal** _____

Nearest; closer to any point of reference; opposite of distal. (The shoulder is distal to the wrist but proximal to the elbow.)

10. **sagittal** _____

Division of body into left and right sides in a vertical lengthwise fashion.

11. **superior** _____

Situated above, or directed upward; in official anatomic nomenclature, used in reference to the upper surface of an organ or other structure, or to a structure occupying a higher position.

12. **transverse** _____

A horizontal plane situated at right angles to the long axis, or sagittal and coronal planes; placed crosswise.

13. **ventral** _____

Pertaining to the abdomen; used to denote a position that is more toward the belly/abdominal surface than some other object of reference.

II. **MULTIPLE CHOICE.**
    Choose the best answer.

1. Placed crosswise.

    ○ coronal
    ○ sagittal
    ○ transverse
    ○ ventral

2. Denoting the lower of two structures.

    ○ inferior
    ○ superior
    ○ sagittal
    ○ coronal

3. Pertaining to the belly-side or the abdomen.

    ○ posterior
    ○ ventral
    ○ inferior
    ○ superior

4. Situated in front of.

   ○ inferior

   ○ transverse

   ○ coronal

   ○ anterior

5. Means to the side.

   ○ medial

   ○ lateral

   ○ inferior

   ○ anterior

6. The farthest point.

   ○ distal

   ○ inferior

   ○ transverse

   ○ medial

7. Nearest.

   ○ distal

   ○ inferior

   ○ lateral

   ○ proximal

8. Pertaining to the middle layer.

   ○ medial

   ○ lateral

   ○ inferior

   ○ posterior

9. Pertaining to the head or crown.

   ○ coronal

   ○ inferior

   ○ superior

   ○ transverse

10. Pertaining to the back.

   ○ dorsal

   ○ superior

   ○ inferior

   ○ ventral

11. Toward the belly surface.

○ coronal

○ sagittal

○ ventral

○ inferior

12. Also pertaining to the back.

○ posterior

○ coronal

○ sagittal

○ ventral

Combining Planes

Term	Combining Form	Examples
anterior	antero	anteroinferior anterolateral anteromedial anteroposterior
distal	disto	distobuccal distocervical distolabial
dorsal	dorso*	dorsoanterior dorsolateral dorsomedial dorsoposterior
inferior	infero	inferolateral inferomedial inferoposterior
lateral	latero	lateroposition lateroversion
medial	medio	mediocarpal mediolateral
posterior	postero	posteroinferior posterolateral posteromedial
superior	supero	superolateral superomedial
ventral	ventro*	ventrodorsal ventrolateral ventroposterior

*dorso- and ventro- can be designed dorsi- and ventri- in certain instances. However, these forms are generally not used in combination with other positional or anatomical planes. Examples would be dorsiflexion and ventriflexion (which mean bending towards the extensor surface of a limb and bending toward the belly, respectively).

Notice that several of the terms can be combined in both directions, such as *inferoposterior* and *posteroinferior*.

It is often the case that a structure (or a mass) being referred to is not found precisely in one plane or direction (e.g., anterior or lateral). Instead, the reference is to somewhere between two different planes or directions. In these instances, it is necessary to combine the planes or directions into one word to describe the location (e.g., anterolateral).

You learned in the Medical Word Building portion of Medical Terminology how to use combining forms. To join directional and positional adjectives, use the combining vowel.

I. **FILL IN THE BLANK.**
    Combine the following directional and positional adjectives.

1. ventral + lateral = _____

2. inferior + posterior = _____

3. posterior + inferior = _____

4. superior + lateral = _____

5. lateral + posterior = _____

6. medial + lateral = _____

7. inferior + medial = _____

8. superior + inferior = _____

9. anterior + medial = _____

10. dorsal + flexion = _____

11. distal + cervical = _____

12. anterior + lateral = _____

Muscles of the Face and Head

You will see these directional components incorporated into the names of a number of muscles. The following figures are provided as a visual guide. Concentrate on body placement of the various muscle groups. We will start at the head and work our way down.

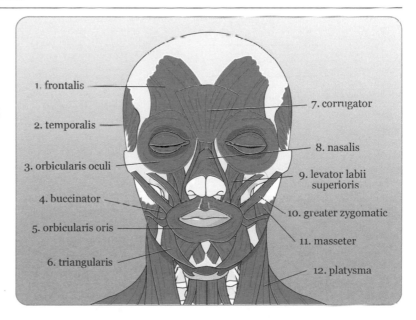

1. frontalis
2. temporalis
3. orbicularis oculi
4. buccinator
5. orbicularis oris
6. triangularis
7. corrugator
8. nasalis
9. levator labii superioris
10. greater zygomatic
11. masseter
12. platysma

I. FILL IN THE BLANK.

In the blanks provided below, refer to the above diagram and enter the term corresponding to the following numbers. Use the word(s) in the box to fill in the blanks.

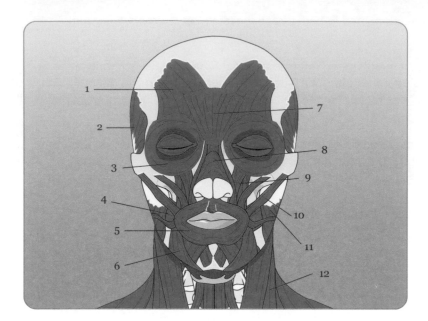

1. _____

2. _____

3. _____

4. _____

5. _____

6. _____

7. _____

8. _____

9. _____

10. _____

11. _____

12. _____

greater zygomatic
buccinator
orbicularis oculi
levator labii superioris
orbicularis oris
masseter
frontalis
platysma
corrugator
temporalis
nasalis
triangularis

II. MULTIPLE CHOICE.
Choose the best answer.

1. The muscle surrounding the eye.
   - ○ frontalis
   - ○ orbicularis oris
   - ○ orbicularis oculi
   - ○ masseter

2. Lower jaw muscle in the shape of a triangle.
   - ○ triangularis
   - ○ temporalis
   - ○ platysma
   - ○ frontalis

3. Muscle located above the eye.
   - ○ buccinator
   - ○ corrugator
   - ○ frontalis
   - ○ temporalis

4. Muscle that runs from the lower jaw down the neck.
   - ○ platysma
   - ○ levator labii superioris
   - ○ greater zygomatic
   - ○ triangularis

5. Cheek muscle.
   - ○ platysma
   - ○ temporalis
   - ○ masseter
   - ○ buccinator

6. Muscle found in the nose.
   - ○ corrugator
   - ○ nasalis
   - ○ platysma
   - ○ greater zygomatic

7. A muscle that lifts and is above the lips.
   - ○ nasalis
   - ○ buccinator
   - ○ orbicularis oris
   - ○ levator labii superioris

8. Muscle surrounding the mouth.
   - ○ orbicularis oris
   - ○ orbicularis oral
   - ○ orbicularis oculi
   - ○ triangularis

9. Muscle found in the lower jaw.
   - ○ buccinator
   - ○ masseter
   - ○ triangularis
   - ○ massiter

10. The larger of the zygomaticus muscles.
    - ○ lesser zygomatic
    - ○ greater zygoma
    - ○ greater zygomatic
    - ○ platysma

11. Muscle located on the side of the head, just above both ears.
    - ○ frontalis
    - ○ temporalis
    - ○ corrugator
    - ○ nasalis

12. Muscle located on the forehead; it creates the "worry lines" or wrinkling of the brow associated with frowning.
    - ○ corrugator
    - ○ corugator
    - ○ corrugater
    - ○ currogator

Muscles of Facial Expression and Mastication

I. **TERMINOLOGY.**
    Enter each term in the space provided. Read the definition and description for each term.

1. **lateral pterygoid** _____

This is a muscle of mastication. It originates on the pterygoid process of the sphenoid bone. It moves the mandible and limits sideways jaw movement.

2. **medial pterygoid** _____

Also a muscle of mastication. Both pterygoid muscles are on the inside of the mandible. The medial pterygoid elevates the jaw and provides sideways jaw movement.

3. **risorius** _____

The risorius originates on the side of the face and inserts on the orbicularis oris muscle. It draws the angle of the mouth laterally (to the side) and enables the human being to smile.

4. **mentalis** _____

The mentalis muscle originates on the chin and goes into the orbicularis oris muscle. It elevates and protrudes the lower lip. Basically it allows for pouting.

5. **depressor labii Inferioris** _____

This muscle also originates on the mandible and inserts on to the orbicularis muscle. It depresses the bottom lip.
(Names: depressor=depress, labii=lips, inferioris=below or bottom)

6. **depressor anguli oris** _____

This muscle originates on the lower part of the mandible. It pulls down the angle of the mouth.
(Names: depressor=depress, anguli=angle, oris=mouth)

SPELLING.
Determine if the following words are spelled correctly. If the spelling is correct, leave the word as it has already been entered. If the spelling is incorrect, provide the correct spelling.

1. mentalis _____   2. depressor _____

3. terygoid _____   4. labi _____

5. risorius _____   6. angguli _____

7. inferioris _____

Muscles of the Neck

Muscles of the neck are used to support and move the head. They are also associated with structures found in the neck region, such as the hyoid bone and the larynx. (The larynx is made up of muscle and cartilage that both guard the entrance to the trachea and the "voice box." It will be discussed in a later unit.)

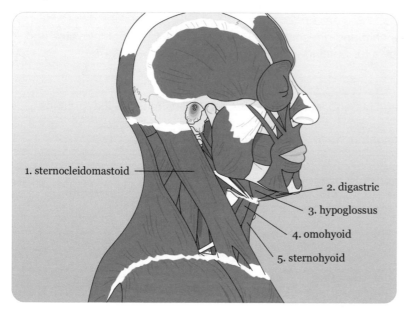

1. sternocleidomastoid

2. digastric

3. hypoglossus

4. omohyoid

5. sternohyoid

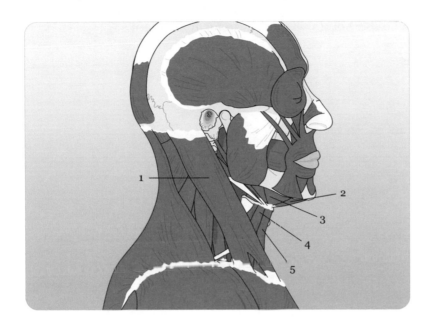

1. _____

2. _____

3. _____

4. _____

5. _____

hyoglossus
sternohyoid
digastric
sternocleidomastoid
omohyoid

Muscles of the Anterior Torso

The linea alba and umbilicus are labeled in the above figure; however, they are not muscles. We have included them here for you to identify where they are. Linea alba means literally "white line" and is the term for the tendinous line down the middle of the anterior abdominal wall directly between the two rectus muscles. The umbilicus, as annotated, is the belly button.

The muscles and terms found on the above figure are for the superficial muscles of the torso only. There are many additional muscles located in this region of the body. If you come across a term that is not delineated above, look in your medical dictionary to find it. The

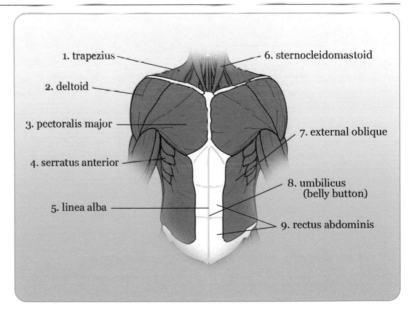

1. trapezius
2. deltoid
3. pectoralis major
4. serratus anterior
5. linea alba
6. sternocleidomastoid
7. external oblique
8. umbilicus (belly button)
9. rectus abdominis

sternocleidomastoid muscle is a muscle of the neck as shown on the previous page. It is shown here for reference only.

I. **FILL IN THE BLANK.**
    Refer to the figure below and use the word(s) in the box to fill in the blanks.

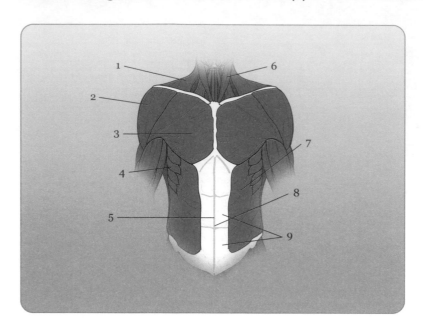

1. _____

2. _____

3. _____

4. _____

5. _____

6. _____

7. _____

8. _____

9. _____

| sternocleidomastoid |
| rectus abdominis |
| serratus anterior |
| pectoralis major |
| external oblique |
| deltoid |
| umbilicus (belly button) |
| linea alba |
| trapezius |

Muscles of the Posterior Torso

As with the earlier figures, these are not all the muscles of the back. These are the superficial ones, and they are the most commonly dictated terms. Notice the term *lumbar aponeurosis*. This is not a muscle. An aponeurosis, as previously stated, is a white, flattened tendinous expansion, serving mainly to connect a muscle with the parts that it moves. It replaces what were formerly called fasciae (plural), although some doctors and dictators may still use the old terminology. Both names are illustrated above.

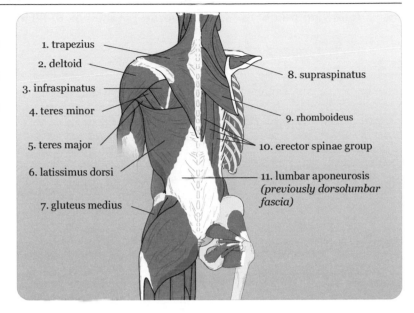

1. trapezius
2. deltoid
3. infraspinatus
4. teres minor
5. teres major
6. latissimus dorsi
7. gluteus medius
8. supraspinatus
9. rhomboideus
10. erector spinae group
11. lumbar aponeurosis *(previously dorsolumbar fascia)*

I. FILL IN THE BLANK.
In the blanks provided below, refer to the figure and enter the term that corresponds to the following numbers. Use the word(s) in the box to fill in the blanks.

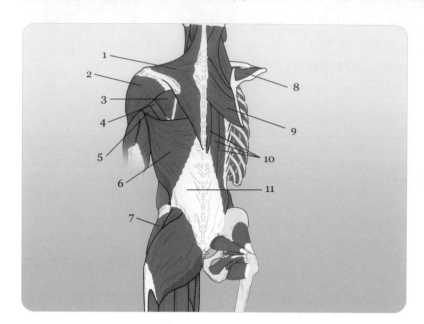

1. _____

2. _____

3. _____

4. _____

5. _____

6. _____

7. _____

8. _____

9. _____

10. _____

11. _____

erector spinae group
teres major
lumbar aponeurosis
infraspinatus
gluteus medius
trapezius
supraspinatus
teres minor
latissimus dorsi
deltoid
rhomboideus (major)

Muscles of the Arm

Thenar is a term that refers to the "mound on the palm at the base of the thumb" and also "pertaining to the palm." The terms *hypothenar* and *thenar* muscles simply describe the location of the muscles and are not the name of individual muscles. You should be able to recognize several muscle names in the arm that are descriptive—terms such as *longus* and *brevis* (long and short) and *radialis* and *ulnaris* (for the radius and ulna bones). In addition, some of these muscles should be easy because they are so commonly known (like the biceps and triceps).

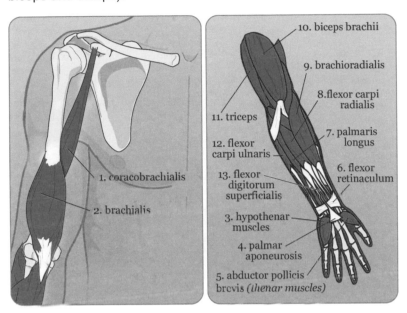

10. biceps brachii
9. brachioradialis
8. flexor carpi radialis
11. triceps
7. palmaris longus
12. flexor carpi ulnaris
6. flexor retinaculum
13. flexor digitorum superficialis
1. coracobrachialis
2. brachialis
3. hypothenar muscles
4. palmar aponeurosis
5. abductor pollicis brevis (*thenar muscles*)

Note the term *flexor retinaculum*. A retinaculum (plural: retinacula) is a structure that holds an organ or tissue in place. (In surgery, it is also used to describe an instrument that retracts tissues.) As with the aponeurosis, this is not a muscle. It is, however, a significant structure of the arm, and it is important in the musculoskeletal system.

It may be helpful to start looking for consistencies in spelling of muscle terms that would make it easier to remember them. For example, the bones of the forearm are the radius and ulna. The muscles that attach to these bones are named for them (radialis, ulnaris, and brachioradialis). All of these terms end in *is*. Look for these similarities and use them as tools for learning the terms.

You will discover that many muscles (although not all of them) end in *is*. It may be easier to learn the exceptions than to memorize each individual term. Of course, if you happened to study Latin along the way, these terms will be simple to learn.

Another feature of muscle terms is that some of them end in *s* but are not plural. There is no such word as *bicep* or *tricep*. The actual definitions for *biceps* and *triceps* are literally muscles with two and three heads, respectively.

I. FILL IN THE BLANK.

In the blanks provided below, refer to the figure and enter the term that corresponds to the following numbers. Use the word(s) in the box to fill in the blanks.

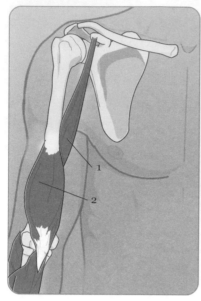 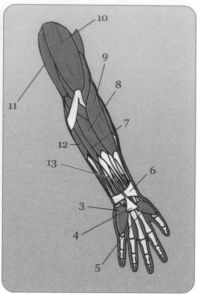

1. _____

2. _____

3. _____

4. _____

5. _____

6. _____

7. _____

8. _____

9. _____

10. _____

11. _____

12. _____

13. _____

flexor retinaculum
brachioradialis
coracobrachialis
abductor pollicis brevis
flexor carpi ulnaris
hypothenar muscles
palmaris longus
brachialis
triceps
biceps brachii
palmar aponeurosis
flexor carpi radialis
flexor digitorum superficialis

Deep Muscles of the Arm

While we have focused mainly on the superficial muscles of the arm, there are other muscles (besides the coracobrachialis and the brachialis) that are located deep in relation to the ones in the figure. Direct your attention to the term *pollicis*. This is derived from the word *pollex*, which means the first digit of the hand (or, more commonly, the thumb). The muscles that act to move the thumb contain the term *pollicis*. In addition to the abductor pollicis brevis, there is an adductor pollicis, an extensor pollicis, and so on. If you can remember that *pollex* means thumb, you can be sure to use *pollicis* in reference to certain muscles in the hand.

When you learn the muscles of the leg you will see the term *hallux*, which is the great toe (or, more commonly, the big toe.) Muscles that act to move the big toe are denoted by the term *hallucis* (derived from *hallux*). As with *carpals/metacarpals* and *tarsals/metatarsals*, it is easy to confuse the terms *hallux* and *pollex* (and likewise *hallucis* and *pollicis*). Learn the root terms, and it will be easier to differentiate between the two words and be certain the right one is being used.

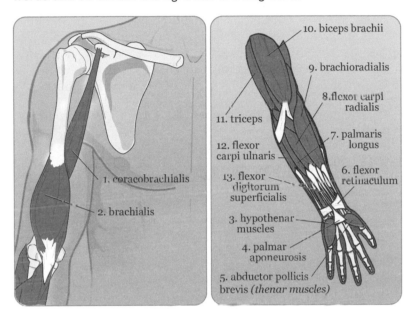

10. biceps brachii
9. brachioradialis
8. flexor carpi radialis
11. triceps
7. palmaris longus
12. flexor carpi ulnaris
6. flexor retinaculum
13. flexor digitorum superficialis
3. hypothenar muscles
4. palmar aponeurosis
5. abductor pollicis brevis *(thenar muscles)*
1. coracobrachialis
2. brachialis

I. **TRUE/FALSE.**
   Mark the following truc or false.

1. Hallucis are the muscles that move the thumb.

   ○ true
   ○ false

2. Pollicis is derived from the word pollex.

   ○ true
   ○ false

3. The pollicis and hallucis are deep, not superficial, muscles.

○ true
○ false

4. Hallux is a word that means the first digit of the hand.

○ true
○ false

Actions of Arm Muscles

The arm and hand muscles are most commonly seen in radiology (x-ray) reports, orthopedics (especially operative notes), and physical therapy, although, as with other terms, they might turn up virtually anywhere. It is important for you to begin to recognize the terms for the muscles associated with the hand that indicate position and movement, as well as more basic body location: supinate, pronate, flex, extend, digits, pollex, for example. The more you understand what you are reading, the more accurate and professional your work will eventually be. Lucky for you, you do **not** have to memorize exactly what each one of these muscles does.

The following are a few of the muscles that are located beneath the muscles shown in the previous figures.

I. **TERMINOLOGY.**
   Enter each term in the space provided. Read the definition and description for each term.

   1. **anconeus** _____

   Located on the back of the humerus, it extends the forearm.

   2. **extensor digiti minimi** _____

   A long narrow muscle located on the ulnar side of the extensor digitorum communis muscle. It assists in extension of the wrist and little finger.

   3. **extensor digitorum communis** _____

   Positioned in the center of the forearm along the posterior surface. Its tendon divides into four tendons beneath the extensor retinaculum, which attach to the distal tips of fingers one through four.

   4. **flexor digitorum profundus** _____

   Lies just underneath the flexor digitorum superficialis muscle. This muscle flexes the distal ends of the fingers (but not the thumb).

   5. **flexor pollicis longus** _____

   Positioned deep on the front of the radius. It attaches at the base of the thumb and flexes the thumb and makes grasping possible.

   6. **pronator teres** _____

   Positioned in upper middle part of the forearm. It arises from the **epicondyle** (a prominence or projection on a bone). It turns the hand downwards (called pronation) and flexes the elbow.

   7. **epicondyle** _____

   A prominence or projection on a bone.

8. **pronator quadratus** _____

Positioned deep and extends between the ulna and radius. It works with the other pronator muscle to rotate the palm of the hand down, as well as position the thumb medially.

9. **supinator** _____

Positioned around the upper portion of the radius. It works with the biceps to turn the palm upwards (called supination).

II. MULTIPLE CHOICE.
Choose the term which best describes the statement.

1. To extend the palm upwards.
   - ○ suppinate
   - ○ supinate
   - ○ pronate
   - ○ suepinate

2. The first digit of the hand (the thumb).
   - ○ hallux
   - ○ polex
   - ○ pollex
   - ○ carpals

3. Located behind the humerus and extends the forearm.
   - ○ anconeus
   - ○ anconius
   - ○ anconeis
   - ○ anconncus

4. Long narrow muscle which assists in extension of the wrist and little finger.
   - ○ extensor digitus minimus
   - ○ extensor digiti minimi
   - ○ extensor digiti mirnini
   - ○ extensor digitus maximus

5. Another term for palmar.
   - ○ tenar
   - ○ theno
   - ○ thenar
   - ○ thennar

6. Descriptive muscle term meaning short.

    ○ longus
    ○ brevus
    ○ brives
    ○ brevis

7. Muscle attached to the humerus deep to the biceps.

    ○ coracobrachialis
    ○ coracobrachialus
    ○ coronobrachialis
    ○ chorobrachialis

8. A structure which holds an organ or a tissue in place.

    ○ aponeurosis
    ○ retinaculum
    ○ retinaculim
    ○ apponeurosis

9. The major muscle of the upper arm.

    ○ bicep
    ○ flexor carpi ulnaris
    ○ biceps
    ○ bicepps

10. A muscle which turns the palm of the hand downwards.

    ○ pronater teres
    ○ pronator teres
    ○ pronator terres
    ○ pronater teris

11. A muscle whose tendon divides into four different tendons.

    ○ extensor digitorum comminus
    ○ extensor digiti comminus
    ○ extensor digitorum communis
    ○ extensor digiti communis

12. Long slender arm muscle with a tendon which attaches to the palmar aponeurosis.

    ○ palmaris longus
    ○ palmaris brevis
    ○ palmarus longis
    ○ palmaris longis

13. Muscle located on the back of the arm.
   - ○ tricep
   - ○ thenar muscle
   - ○ bicep
   - ○ triceps

14. Muscle which flexes the fingers.
   - ○ flesor digitorum profundis
   - ○ flexor digitorum profundus
   - ○ extensor digiti profundidi
   - ○ flexor digotorum profundus

Muscles of the Leg

The femur is the longest and strongest bone in the body and, correspondingly, the muscles of the legs represent some of the longest and strongest muscles.

There are also a few terms listed on this image (and subsequent images) that are not muscles, although they are vital to the musculoskeletal system—especially the lower extremities. Notice the calcaneal or Achilles tendon. The Achilles is the thickest and strongest tendon in the body. You have already learned that tendons are fibrous cords to which muscle is attached.

If you are into mythology, you may know that the Achilles tendon is named for the Greek fighter Achilles. He was immortal and invulnerable except for the spot on his heel where he was held as he was dipped into the river water that turns mortals into gods. It was this area that was pierced by an arrow during the Trojan War, and this wound caused his death.

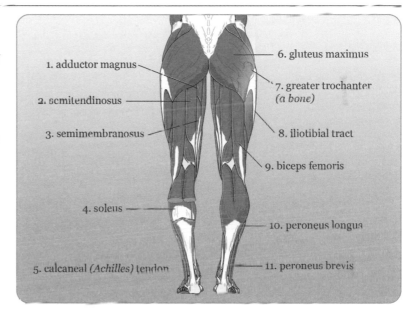

1. adductor magnus
2. semitendinosus
3. semimembranosus
4. soleus
5. calcaneal (*Achilles*) tendon
6. gluteus maximus
7. greater trochanter (*a bone*)
8. iliotibial tract
9. biceps femoris
10. peroneus longus
11. peroneus brevis

The extensor retinaculum is not a muscle but covers and holds in place the muscles and tendons of the front of the foot. The greater trochanter, also called trochanter major, is a broad, flat process to which several muscles are attached. Finally, the iliotibial tract is a thick, long band of fascia lata that extends down the side of the thigh to the tibia.

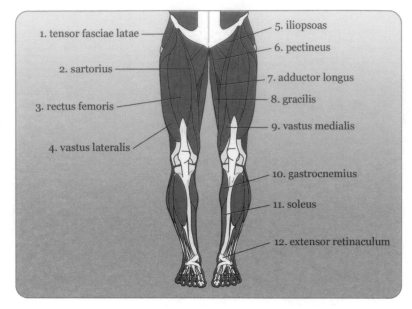

1. tensor fasciae latae
2. sartorius
3. rectus femoris
4. vastus lateralis
5. iliopsoas
6. pectineus
7. adductor longus
8. gracilis
9. vastus medialis
10. gastrocnemius
11. soleus
12. extensor retinaculum

I. FILL IN THE BLANK.

In the blanks provided below, refer to the image and enter the terms that correspond to the following numbers. Use the words in the box to fill in the blanks.

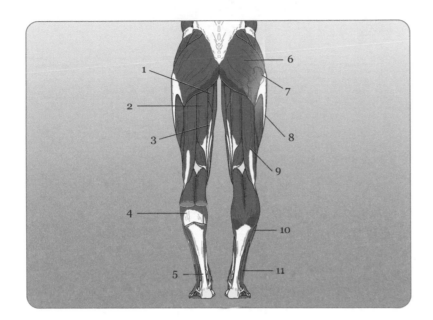

1. _____

2. _____

3. _____

4. _____

5. _____

6. _____

7. _____

8. _____

9. _____

10. _____

11. _____

iliotibial tract
semimembranosus
peroneus brevis
adductor magnus
gluteus maximus
semitendinosus
peroneus longus
biceps femoris
greater trochanter
soleus
calcaneal (Achilles) tendon

II. FILL IN THE BLANK.

In the blanks provided below, refer to the image and enter the terms that correspond to the following numbers. Use the words in the box to fill in the blanks.

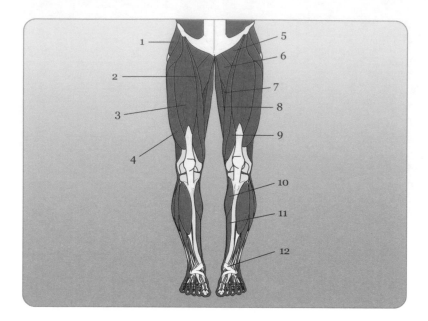

1. _____

2. _____

3. _____

4. _____

5. _____

6. _____

7. _____

8. _____

9. _____

10. _____

11. _____

12. _____

adductor longus
sartorius
gastrocnemius
rectus femoris
vastus medialis
iliopsoas
extensor retinaculum
soleus
pectineus
tensor fasciae latae
gracilis
vastus lateralis

Muscles of the Lower Leg

The lateral malleolus is another term that is not a muscle but is important to the musculoskeletal system. *Lateral*, of course, means side, and a *malleolus* is a part of a bone. The lateral malleolus is the bony protuberance found on the lateral side of the ankle joint. The medial malleolus is likewise a bony protuberance, but it is found on the medial side of the joint.

Incidentally, in medical notes, the legs are rarely referred to as "legs." They are instead called the lower extremities. (The arms are likewise called the upper extremities). An extremity is simply the name for a limb. You should notice, as with the arm muscles, that there are several descriptive terms in the graphics

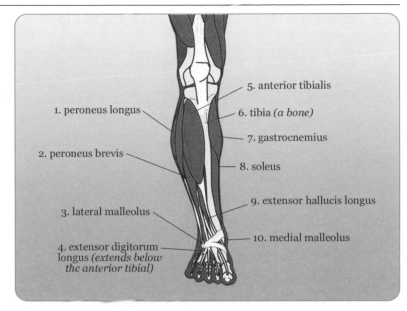

1. peroneus longus

2. peroneus brevis

3. lateral malleolus

4. extensor digitorum longus *(extends below the anterior tibial)*

5. anterior tibialis

6. tibia *(a bone)*

7. gastrocnemius

8. soleus

9. extensor hallucis longus

10. medial malleolus

which should be familiar by now, such as *longus, brevis, hallucis*, and *maximus*. Take just a moment to find any terms that you already know.

I. FILL IN THE BLANK.

In the blanks provided below, refer to the image and enter the terms that correspond to the following numbers. Use the words in the box to fill in the blanks.

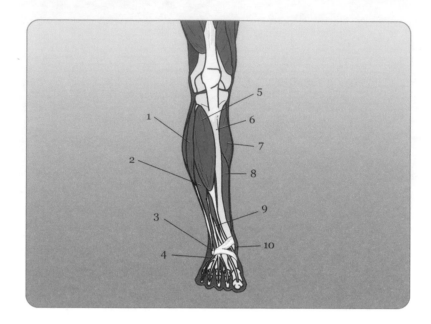

1. _____

2. _____

3. _____

4. _____

5. _____

6. _____

7. _____

8. _____

9. _____

10. _____

extensor digitorum longus
gastrocnemius
peroneus longus
medial malleolus
lateral malleolus
extensor hallucis longus
anterior tibialis
soleus
tibia
peroneus brevis

Review: Muscle Anatomy

As with any other part of the human anatomy, there are several things that can go wrong with these structures. Before you begin learning about pertinent disease processes, review all of the muscle groups that you have studied. Do the exercises on the following pages, and remember that the answers could be from any of the figures found in the muscle lessons.

I. FILL IN THE BLANK.
Determine which part of the body the muscle or term is part of (back, arm, leg, neck, torso, face).

1. _____ mentalis

2. _____ flexor carpi ulnaris

3. _____ gluteus maximus

4. _____ buccinator

5. _____ sternocleidomastoid

6. _____ temporalis

7. _____ biceps

8. _____ latissimus dorsi

9. _____ orbicularis oris

10. _____ risorius

11. _____ anconeus

12. _____ palmaris longus

13. _____ trapezius

14. _____ platysma

15. _____ digastric

16. _____ brachioradialis

17. _____ supinator

18. _____ corrugator

19. _____ teres major

20. _____ peroneus longus

21. _____ gracilis

22. _____ nasalis

23. _____ lateral malleolus

24. _____ brachialis

25. _____ labii inferioris

26. _____ medial pterygoid

27. _____ soleus

28. _____ masseter

29. _____ adductor magnus

30. _____ serratus anterior

31. _____ omohyoid

32. _____ pronator teres

33. _____ tensor fasciae latae

34. _____ iliopsoas

35. _____ greater zygomatic

36. _____ anterior tibia

37. _____ greater trochanter

38. _____ supraspinatus

39. _____ depressor anguli oris

40. _____ external oblique

41. _____ extensor digiti minimi

42. _____ lumbar aponeurosis

43. _____ gastrocnemius

II. MULTIPLE CHOICE.
Choose the best answer.

1. The forearm muscle that pronates the hand.
   - ○ anconeus
   - ○ pronater dupli
   - ○ pronator teres
   - ○ biceps

2. A muscle that has two heads.
   - ○ triceps
   - ○ tricep
   - ○ bicep
   - ○ biceps

3. The muscle that makes pouting possible.
   - ○ mentalis
   - ○ lateral pterygoid
   - ○ linea obliquus
   - ○ frownicus

4. The major muscle of the rear end.
   - ○ gluteus largus
   - ○ gluteus minimus
   - ○ gluteus maximus
   - ○ posteroanterior

5. A long narrow muscle that assists in extending the wrist and little finger.
   - ○ extensor digiti minimus
   - ○ extensor digiti minimi
   - ○ brevis
   - ○ flexorum digiti minimi

6. The long muscle responsible for movement of the big toe.
   - ○ extensor hallucis longus
   - ○ extensor hallucis brevis
   - ○ external oblique
   - ○ mentalis

7. Previously called the dorsolumbar fascia.

   ○ brevis
   ○ lumbar aponeurosis
   ○ flexor retinaculum
   ○ occipitalis

8. Shaped like a rhomboid.

   ○ romboideus
   ○ rhomboidius
   ○ rhombodeus
   ○ rhomboideus

9. The major superficial muscle of the shoulder.

   ○ deltoid
   ○ occipitalis
   ○ gluteus maximus
   ○ biceps

10. Muscles responsible for chewing, located on the mandible.

    ○ lateral and medial pterygoid
    ○ medial pterigoid
    ○ lateral pterigoid
    ○ medial and lateral pterigoid

11. Bony prominence on the side of the ankle joint.

    ○ superior malleolus
    ○ lateral malleolus
    ○ greater trochanter
    ○ Achilles tendon

12. The muscle above the lips that is responsible for lifting.

    ○ platysma
    ○ costovertebral
    ○ levator labii superioris
    ○ biceps femoris

13. A muscle with three heads.

    ○ biceps
    ○ bicep
    ○ tricep
    ○ triceps

14. Abdominal muscle.

   ◯ external oblique
   ◯ external abdominis
   ◯ Achilles tendon
   ◯ linea oblique

15. Muscle surrounding the mouth.

   ◯ orbicularis oris
   ◯ costovertebral
   ◯ boca muscalis
   ◯ gracillus

16. Tendon named for a Greek hero.

   ◯ Hercules tendon
   ◯ Achilles tendon
   ◯ Archimedes tendon
   ◯ Zeus tendon

17. Process on the outer thigh to which several muscles are attached.

   ◯ lesser trochanter
   ◯ gluteus maximus
   ◯ greater trochanter
   ◯ gluteus minimus

18. Above and to the side.

   ◯ distolateral
   ◯ lateroventricular
   ◯ inferolateral
   ◯ superolateral

19. Muscle of the back of the leg.

   ◯ gluteus maximus
   ◯ semimembranosus
   ◯ gluteus minimus
   ◯ propioception

20. The term for perception of the stimuli.

   ◯ mentalis
   ◯ gracilis
   ◯ proprioception
   ◯ proprietor

21. The muscle that extends diagonally across the forearm and inserts onto the base of the second and third metacarpal bones.

   ○ flexor carpi radialis
   ○ flexor biceps radialis
   ○ biceps femoris
   ○ linea oblique

22. This is the most superficial of the medial thigh muscles.

   ○ levator labii superioris
   ○ gracilis
   ○ longus
   ○ brevis

23. This muscle can extend, laterally rotate, and adduct the thigh, as well as flex the knee.

   ○ biceps femoris
   ○ triceps femoris
   ○ biceps brevis
   ○ triceps brevis

24. Not the largest or the smallest of the gluteal muscles.

   ○ gluteus medius
   ○ gluteus maximus
   ○ gluteus chica
   ○ gluteus minimus

25. Term meaning short.

   ○ brevus
   ○ brevis
   ○ longus
   ○ longis

26. The system to which muscles belong.

   ○ muculoskeletal system
   ○ musculoskelletal system
   ○ circulatory system
   ○ musculoskeletal system

27. From back to front.

   ○ posteroanterior
   ○ spinofrontalis
   ○ ventrolateral
   ○ costovertebral

Muscular Diseases

As with any other part of the human anatomy, the muscles, their attachments, and associated structures can be injured, infected, diseased, or deformed. Minor muscle injuries are usually diagnosed and treated by family practice doctors. They are also routinely treated in emergency rooms and clinics. However, more serious injuries or disease processes affecting the muscles will be managed by orthopedists and orthopedic surgeons.

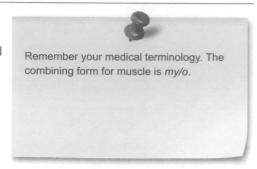

Remember your medical terminology. The combining form for muscle is *my/o*.

These are the specialties where processes involving the muscles will be seen most often. However, people with multiple medical problems across several specialties may be treated for muscle abnormalities in some other specialties (e.g., neurology) as well.

There are literally hundreds of problems that can affect the muscles and/or the musculoskeletal system. Virtually every muscle has a different name for the specific type of injury that could occur to it. Because of the sheer volume of these individual processes, we will be focusing on more general problems and the most common injuries that afflict muscles. If necessary, any individual term can be referenced in a medical dictionary.

Many of the disease processes are created with the combining forms you learned in Medical Word Building. For example, the combining form for muscle is *my/o*. The suffix that means pain is *-algia*. Therefore, muscle pain is called myalgia.

Several brain functions or neurological problems manifest themselves through the muscles, taking the form of abnormal muscular movements. For example, a seizure is a sudden attack of a disease, but is commonly thought of in reference to epilepsy. Epilepsy is any of a group of syndromes that are characterized by a disturbance in brain function that results in loss of consciousness, abnormal motor phenomena, or neurosensory disturbances. An episode resulting from an epileptic condition is called a seizure.

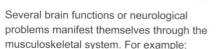

Highlights

Several brain functions or neurological problems manifest themselves through the musculoskeletal system. For example:

- **Epilepsy** – tonic/clonic activity
- **Parkinson disease** – muscular rigidity; muscle tremors

The "abnormal motor phenomena" are manifested in the muscular system. A common type of abnormal motor activity is clonic activity. *Clonic* is the adjectival form of *clonus*, which means alternate muscular contraction and relaxation in rapid succession. It is a term generally used in conjunction with the term *tonic*, which means normal tone. So during a seizure it is often the case that the muscles go through a series of rapid contractions alternating with a return to normal muscle tone. This movement is called tonic/clonic activity or tonicoclonic activity. Although it is not actually caused by an injury to—or defect in—the muscles themselves, it undoubtedly affects the muscular system.

Another common neurologic disorder that affects the muscular system is Parkinson disease. This is a progressive degenerative nervous system disorder that is characterized by four features: slowness and absence of movement, muscular rigidity, resting tremor, and unstable posture. Rigidity means stiffness or inflexibility. This is the fourth most common disease afflicting the elderly. Again, while the cause of the disorder is neurological, all of the manifestations are musculoskeletal.

MULTIPLE CHOICE.
Choose the best answer.

1. Serious muscle injuries or diseases will be managed by _____.

   ○ family practice doctors
   ○ instant care clinics
   ○ orthopedists
   ○ orthopods

2. An epileptic episode resulting in a loss of consciousness, abnormal motor phenomena, or neurosensory disturbances is most commonly called _____.

   ○ a seizure
   ○ an epileptic attack
   ○ a myalgia
   ○ passing out

3. Alternate muscular contraction and relaxation in rapid succession is called _____.

   ○ epilepsy
   ○ myalgia
   ○ tonic activity
   ○ clonic activity

4. The cause of Parkinson disease is _____.

   ○ neurological
   ○ muskuloskeletal
   ○ neurological, but manifests in the musculoskeletal system
   ○ muskuloskeletal, but manifests in the neurological system

Disease Terminology – Lesson 1

I. **TERMINOLOGY.**
Enter each term in the space provided. Read the definition and description for each term.

1. **atony** _____

Lack of normal tone or strength. This happens in muscles that are deprived of innervation (which is the supply of nerve fibers functionally connected with a part). Try not to confuse this term with atrophy (below) or atopy (which is a genetic predisposition towards hypersensitivity to common environmental antigens).

2. **atrophy** _____

The wasting away or weakening of muscle fibers due to a lack of usage. There are many different kinds of atrophy. Look up "atrophy" in a medical dictionary and read or scan the terms that appear under this category.

3. **bursitis** _____

Inflammation of a bursa.

4. **bursa** _____

A sac-like cavity filled with synovial fluid and located in places where tendons or muscles pass over bony prominences.

5. **charley horse** _____

A bruised or torn muscle accompanied by cramps and severe pain. This particular injury most commonly affects the quadriceps muscle. (Incidentally, quadriceps is like biceps or triceps, which always ends in -s, whether singular or plural.) Lay people refer to any muscle spasm of the legs or feet as a charley horse.

6. **cramp** _____

A sustained spasm or contraction of a muscle accompanied by severe, localized pain.

7. **dystonia** _____

Sustained abnormal postures or disruptions of normal movement resulting from alterations of muscle tone.

8. **Dupuytren contracture** _____

Painless thickening and contracture of the palmar fascia due to fibrous proliferation, resulting in loss of function of the fingers.

9. **fasciculations** _____

Similar to fibrillations or tremors. A repetitive, involuntary contraction of muscle. The main cause is nerve damage.

10. **fibromyalgia** _____

A rheumatic disorder characterized by achy pain, tenderness, and stiffness.

11 **myofascial pain syndrome** _____

Fibromyalgia is also called myofascial pain syndrome and fibromyositis. A group of rheumatic disorders caused by achy pain, tenderness, and stiffness of muscles and tendon insertions.

12. **ganglion** _____

A thin-walled band cyst formed on a joint capsule or tendon sheath.

13. **leiomyoma** _____

A benign tumor of smooth muscle tissue (e.g., the uterus).

14. **muscular dystrophy** _____

A genetic abnormality of muscle tissue characterized by dysfunction and ultimately deterioration.

Disease Terminology – Lesson 2

I. **TERMINOLOGY.**
   Enter each term in the space provided. Read the definition and description for each term.

1. **myalgia** _____

   Muscle pain.

2. **myasthenia gravis** _____

   A chronic progressive neuromuscular weakness, usually starting with the muscles of the face and throat.

3. **myopathy** _____

   Any disease of the muscles.

4. **myositis ossificans** _____

   A disease characterized by bony deposits or the ossification of muscle tissue.

5. **paralysis** _____

   The loss of nervous control of a muscle. Paralysis is commonly thought of as related to paraplegia, a paralysis of the legs (lower extremities) or quadriplegia, a paralysis of all four limbs. However, there are many different types of paralysis affecting many different muscles and organs of the body. These can be seen in a medical dictionary under paralysis.

6. **paraplegia** _____

   A paralysis of the legs (lower extremities).

7. **quadriplegia** _____

   A paralysis of all four limbs.

8. **plantar fasciitis** _____

   Excessive pulling or stretching of the calcaneal periosteum by the plantar fascia, resulting in pain along the inner border of the plantar fascia. This definition applies specifically to the process that affects the plantar surface of the foot. Fasciitis is inflammation of the fascia. There are other types of fasciitis, which can be seen in a medical dictionary under fasciitis.

9. **polymyositis** _____

   An autoimmune disorder which causes atrophy and weakness of the muscles.

10. **rigor mortis** _____

    Rigor means chilled, stiffness, rigidity. Rigor mortis is the muscular hardness occurring 4–7 hours after death.

11. **tendinitis** _____

    Inflammation of tendons and of tendon-muscle attachments due to trauma or repetitive wear. (Note the spelling: tendonitis is an acceptable alternative spelling, but tendinitis is preferred.)

12. **tennis elbow** _____

Also called lateral and medial epicondylitis. A strain of the lateral forearm muscles or the tendinous attachments near their origin on the epicondyle of the humerus. (Again note that when "tendon" is changed to another form, the "o" changes to "i"—tendinous.)

13. **tetanus** _____

A disease caused by the bacterium Clostridium tetani, which produces a toxin that causes muscles to go into tetany (hyperexcitability of nerves and muscles, specifically characterized by muscular cramps and twitching). Jaw muscles are affected first. Lockjaw is the more common name.

14. **torticollis** _____

Persistent contraction of a sternocleidomastoid muscle, drawing the head to one side and distorting the face. Causes rotation of the head.

Unit 5
Digestive System

Digestive System – Introduction

Just as bones and muscles are vital in supporting the human body, nutritious food and fluids are also vital to growth, repair, and production of body energy. The digestive system is the body system through which all consumed liquid and solid materials pass, enabling body organs to absorb and metabolize important nutrients.

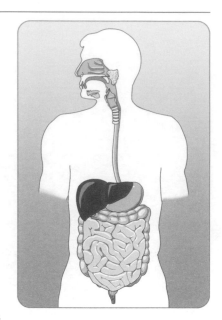

Abdomen refers to the central part of the body from below the chest to the hips. The generic term *gut* is sometimes used as well; however, in medicine this generally refers to the developing GI (gastrointestinal) tract of an embryo. The term *viscera* (singular is *viscus*) is often used to designate the individual organs of digestion; however, the term is actually a general term for any organ of the abdominal or thoracic cavity. This would include digestive organs such as the liver and pancreas, but also respiratory organs such as the lungs. These are not specific medical anatomic terms, but rather a method of designating the external area specific to organs of digestion.

The digestive tract is a tube (lumen) that extends from the mouth to the anus. There are several organ systems connected along this path, such as the gallbladder, liver, pancreas, and salivary glands. Each organ has a specific function vital to the health of the human body, and the nutrients taken in through the digestive process are crucial to their ability to function. In other words, the digestive system consists of all of the parts of the body associated with solids and liquids from entrance by way of the mouth on down until every nutrient has been absorbed and the waste eliminated. Liquid waste is mostly eliminated through the urinary tract system; however, due to its close association with structures of the reproductive system, the urinary system will be introduced in a later unit.

Mouth and Associated Organs

The structure and function of the digestive system begins with the mouth (oral cavity) and its associated organs. Food enters the mouth, is moistened by saliva, is masticated by the teeth, all while being manipulated and tasted by the tongue. The lips (labia) and cheeks hold food in the mouth (which is probably why your parents taught you to chew with your mouth closed).

The oral cavity is divided into two sections: the vestibule and oral cavity proper. With your teeth and mouth shut tight, the vestibule is the space between the teeth and the lips or cheeks, and the oral cavity proper is the space internal to the teeth, where the tongue lies. The lining of the inside of the mouth is made of a stratified squamous epithelium, which protects it from abrasion due to hard or sharp foods during chewing. As you learned in the muscles unit of anatomy, the cheeks are formed by the buccinator muscles (hence the term *buccal* that pertains to the cheeks) and the lips by the orbicularis oris muscle.

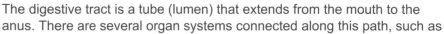

Highlights

The oral cavity is divided into two sections: The vestibule and oral cavity proper.

Vestibule: Space between teeth and lips/cheeks.

Oral Cavity Proper: Space internal to the teeth (where tongue lies).

The part of the lips that we lick the most, where lipstick is applied and kisses are received or given, is called the red margin, with the line between the red of the lips and the skin above is the vermilion border. This is very thin and translucent tissue so the red color is actually derived from blood flow in the underlying capillaries. There are no sweat glands or salivary glands in the red margin of the lips so periodic moistening of the lips by the tongue is needed to prevent drying and cracking. The lip is connected to the inner mucosa of the gum by way of the labial frenulum (which means "little bridle of the lip").

I. FILL IN THE BLANK.
Enter the correct word in the blank provided.

1. Another word for lips, the _____ works with the cheeks to hold food in your mouth.

2. The space between the teeth and the lips or cheeks is called the _____.

3. The _____ is the space internal to the teeth that contains the tongue.

4. The _____ is the lining that protects the inside of the mouth from hard or sharp foods.

5. The area of the lips where lipstick is applied is called the _____.

6. The line between the red of the lips and the skin is called the _____.

7. The lips are connected to the gums with the _____.

Palate

The palate forms the roof of the mouth and is made of two distinct sections, the hard palate and the soft palate. The hard palate is located anteriorly and the soft palate posteriorly. If you take a moment and place the tip of your tongue on the roof of your mouth just behind the teeth and gums and press, you will find the hard palate. The hard palate forms a rigid surface against which the tongue forces food during mastication. Now move your tongue to the back of the roof of your mouth just in front of your uvula and press again; this is the soft palate. The soft palate rises during swallowing to close off the nasopharynx. To see how this functions, try to breathe and swallow at the same time. The uvula is a finger-like piece of soft tissue that hangs down at the opening of the throat. It is anchored to the free edge of the soft palate.

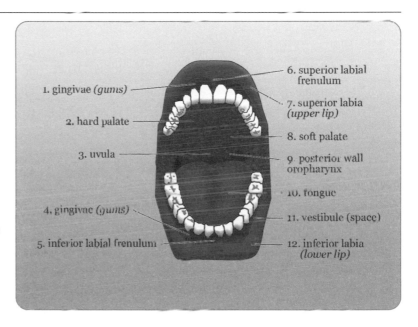

1. gingivae *(gums)*
2. hard palate
3. uvula
4. gingivae *(gums)*
5. inferior labial frenulum
6. superior labial frenulum
7. superior labia *(upper lip)*
8. soft palate
9. posterior wall oropharynx
10. tongue
11. vestibule (space)
12. inferior labia *(lower lip)*

I. FILL IN THE BLANK.
Enter the bolded terms in the space provided.

1. **gingivae** _____

2. **hard palate** _____

3. **inferior labia** _____

4. **inferior labial frenulum** _____

5. **posterior wall oropharynx** _____

6. **soft palate** _____

7. **superior labia** _____

8. **superior labial frenulum** _____

9. **tongue** _____

10. **uvula** _____

11. **vestibule** _____

II. FILL IN THE BLANK.
Refer to the image and enter the term corresponding to the following numbers. Use the words in the box to fill in the blanks.

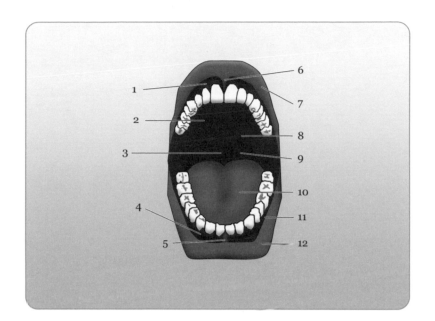

1. _____

2. _____

3. _____

4. _____

5. _____

6. _____

7. _____

8. _____

9. _____

10. _____

11. _____

12. _____

superior labia (upper lip)
gingivae (gums)
soft palate
posterior wall oropharynx
inferior labial frenulum
vestibule
inferior labia (lower lip)
superior labial frenulum
tongue
hard palate
gingivae (gums)
uvula

III. **MULTIPLE CHOICE.**
   Choose the best answer.

   1. Another name for an organ.
      ○ viscera
      ○ lumen
      ○ serosa
      ○ peristalsis

   2. The hollow part of a tube.
      ○ lingual
      ○ perineum
      ○ mesentery
      ○ lumen

   3. Another name for the mouth.
      ○ lingual
      ○ oral cavity
      ○ pharynx
      ○ mucosa

   4. Term that means literally "pertaining to the cheek."
      ○ facial
      ○ alimentary canal
      ○ buccal
      ○ lingual frenulum

   5. Refers to the GI tract of an embryo.
      ○ gut
      ○ abdomen
      ○ tummy
      ○ adventitia

   6. Describes the body from the chest to the hips.
      ○ abdomen
      ○ dorsal mesentery
      ○ retroperitoneal
      ○ viscera

Tongue

The tongue is a muscle that occupies most of the space on the floor of the mouth. The tongue serves several purposes:

- Contains taste buds for the ability to taste food and differentiate between sour, sweet, bitter, and spicy.
- Manipulates food that is being chewed by gripping it and repositioning it between the teeth for mastication.
- Helps mix saliva with food in order to form a compact mass or bolus of food.
- During swallowing, the tongue helps to push the food bolus or liquids into the pharynx for further digestion.
- In speech, the tongue aids in the formation of various consonants, such as d, k, l, n, t, and w.

The tongue is made up of two different types of muscles: extrinsic and intrinsic. Extrinsic muscles allow the tongue to change position, protrude, retract, move laterally, or wiggle. Intrinsic muscles allow the tongue to change shape to flat, round, firm, and relaxed.

Anatomy of the Tongue

The tongue is secured to the floor of the mouth by the lingual frenulum. This secures the tongue into its position and limits its posterior movements so the tongue cannot be easily swallowed. When the lingual frenulum is abnormally short or long, a person is said to be "tongue-tied" (ankyloglossia), which distorts their speech and overly restricts tongue movement. This abnormality is corrected by snipping the lingual frenulum, once again allowing movement of the tongue and improving speech.

The superior surface of the tongue consists of three major types of projections:

1. lingual tonsils
2. circumvallate papillae
3. fungiform papillae (large bumps)
4. epiglottis
5. lingual tonsils
6. sulcus terminalis
7. filiform papillae (small bumps)

- filiform papillae
- fungiform papillae
- circumvallate papillae

The filiform papillae lend a rough surface to the tongue, allowing it to grasp food and manipulate it during mastication. The filiform papillae are very numerous and give the tongue its whitish appearance, lining up in parallel rows.

The fungiform papillae have a vascular core that gives them a reddish appearance. Fungiform papillae, like their name "fungi," actually have a mushroom-like appearance.

Taste buds are located in the epithelium on the tops of fungiform papillae. Take a moment and look into a mirror at your tongue (in a very well lit room), and see if you can see these scattered fungiform papillae on the surface of your tongue. They are not as abundant as the filiform papillae but are more visible. As you may know, a swollen taste bud is a very painful and very visible malady that most individuals suffer on occasion.

Two-thirds of the way back on the tongue surface and anterior to the sulcus terminalis (a groove that marks the border between the mouth and the pharynx) lies the circumvallate papillae. There are 10–12 circumvallate papillae that lie in the shape of a V. These are individually surrounded by a circular ridge and the epithelium on the sides of these papillae contain more taste buds.

The posterior third of the tongue, or the root of the tongue, is considered part of the oropharynx and contains lingual tonsils. Many individuals who have had their tonsils surgically removed can continue to get tonsillitis; however, this type of tonsillitis is called lingual tonsillitis and is treated with antibiotics.

I. **FILL IN THE BLANK.**
    Enter the bolded terms in the space provided.

       1. **circumvallate papillae** _____

       2. **epiglottis** _____

       3. **filiform papillae** _____

       4. **fungiform papillae** _____

       5. **lingual tonsils** _____

       6. **sulcus terminalis** _____

II. FILL IN THE BLANK.
Refer to the image and enter the term corresponding to the following numbers. Use the words in the box to fill in the blanks.

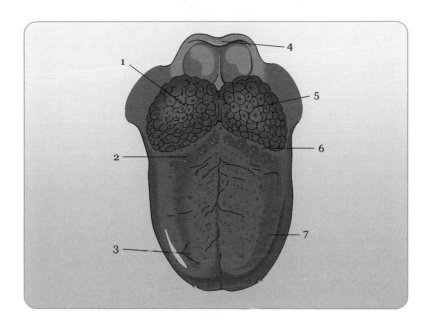

1. _____

2. _____

3. _____

4. _____

5. _____

6. _____

7. _____

sulcus terminalis
lingual tonsils
filiform papillae
circumvallate papillae
lingual tonsils
epiglottis
fungiform papillae

III. **MULTIPLE CHOICE.**
Choose the best answer.

1. Elevations on the tongue.
   - ○ papillae
   - ○ serosa
   - ○ omentum
   - ○ buccal

2. Means pertaining to the tongue.
   - ○ inguinal
   - ○ oral
   - ○ buccal
   - ○ lingual

3. The tongue is connected to the floor of the mouth via the _____.
   - ○ lingual frenulum
   - ○ buccal
   - ○ oral cavity
   - ○ muscularis

Salivary Glands

Salivary glands produce saliva, which is a complex mixture of water, ions, mucus, and enzymes. This complex contains a bicarbonate buffer that neutralizes bacteria-producing acids to help prevent tooth decay, provides proteins that stimulate the growth of good bacteria, and contains antiviral substances, antibodies, and a cyanide compound, which kills harmful microorganisms.

Saliva moistens the mouth, dissolves food, wets food, and binds it into a bolus, allowing the enzymes in the saliva to start the digestive process before food is propelled towards the alimentary canal.

> **Highlights**
>
> Saliva moistens the mouth, dissolves food, wets food, and binds it into a bolus, allowing the enzymes in the saliva to start the digestive process before food is propelled towards the alimentary canal.

There are two distinct types of salivary glands: small intrinsic salivary glands, and large extrinsic salivary glands.

The small intrinsic salivary glands are located throughout the mouth, in the mucosa of the tongue, palate, lips, and cheeks and are responsible for maintaining a moist mouth.

Large extrinsic salivary glands lie external to the mouth, but their ducts connect to it. They secrete saliva only when we eat or when we anticipate eating. There are three pairs of extrinsic salivary glands: parotid, submandibular, and sublingual.

I. MULTIPLE CHOICE.
Choose the best answer.

1. Saliva is a combination of _____.
   - ◯ water, ions, mucus, and enzymes
   - ◯ water, acid, and mucus
   - ◯ mucus and enzymes
   - ◯ water, mucus, and enzymes

2. The proteins in saliva stimulate _____.
   - ◯ digestion
   - ◯ growth of bad bateria
   - ◯ growth of good bacteria
   - ◯ tooth decay

3. Which of the following does the bicarbonate buffer in saliva do?
   - ◯ promotes growth of good bacteria
   - ◯ helps prevent tooth decay
   - ◯ kills harmful microorganisms
   - ◯ all of the above

4. When do large extrinsic salivary glands secrete saliva?
   - ◯ constantly
   - ◯ after we eat
   - ◯ every few hours
   - ◯ when we eat or anticipate eating

5. Where are small intrinsic salivary glands located?
   - ◯ on the tongue, palate, lips, and cheeks
   - ◯ outside the mouth, connected to it by ducts
   - ◯ only on the tongue
   - ◯ on the tongue and cheeks

Teeth

Our teeth allow us to masticate (chew) our food by tearing, grinding, and breaking it into tiny pieces that can then be digested. There are two sets of teeth (dentitions) present at birth. The first set to erupt are the deciduous teeth (baby teeth), followed by the permanent teeth.

Underneath the deciduous teeth lie the permanent teeth. Between the ages of 5–12, the deciduous teeth are reabsorbed until they loosen and fall out.

Teeth fall into four classifications:

1. incisors
2. canines
3. premolars
4. molars

Teeth have different classifications. These classifications are made according to shape and function of the teeth. Teeth fall into four classifications: incisors, canines, premolars, and molars.

Shaped like a chisel, the main function of the incisor is to bite off pieces of food, the canines (eyeteeth/cuspids) pierce and tear food, and premolars (bicuspids) and molars grind and mash food with a tremendous crushing power.

Teeth are surrounded by a pink, fleshy tissue called gingiva (gums). Teeth consist of three main parts: crown, neck, and root.

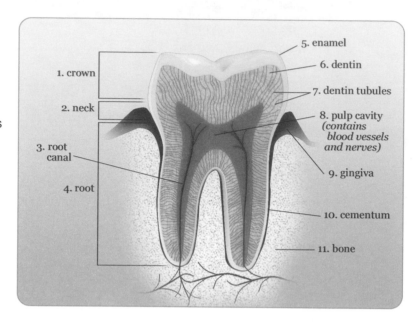

The crown is covered in enamel, which is the hardest substance in the body. It gives the teeth a white appearance and protects them from friction. Beneath the enamel is the dentin. This is considerably softer than enamel and is a yellowish, bony tissue. The innermost part of the tooth is the pulp cavity, which is filled with dental pulp, a loose connective tissue containing the nerve endings and blood vessels. This pulp supplies the tooth with nutrients and sensation. When a tooth is damaged by a blow or by a deep cavity, the pulp may become infected or even die. When this occurs, a root canal procedure must be performed. In this procedure the pulp is drilled out and the pulp cavity is sterilized and filled with a substance before the tooth can be capped.

The protective layer that covers the root is the cementum and the periodontal membrane actually holds the tooth in place. The crown and root meet near the gum line and form what is called the neck of the tooth.

Dental cavities or caries are a result of a gradual deterioration or demineralization of the tooth enamel and dentin due to bacteria. Dental plaque is a buildup of sugar, bacteria, and other debris that adheres to the surface of the teeth. These trapped sugars then metabolize and produce an acid that dissolves the calcium salts within the teeth. When the calcium salts have been leached out of the teeth, protein-digesting enzymes then destroy the remaining tooth matrix. Brushing teeth frequently helps to prevent dental cavities and tooth decay.

I. **FILL IN THE BLANK.**
   Enter the bolded terms in the space provided.

1. **bone** _____   2. **cementum** _____

3. **crown** _____   4. **dentin** _____

5. **dentin tubules** _____   6. **enamel** _____

7. **gingiva** _____   8. **neck** _____

9. **pulp cavity** _____   10. **root** _____

11. **root canal** _____

II. FILL IN THE BLANK.
Refer to the image and enter the term corresponding to the following numbers. Use the words in the box to fill in the blanks.

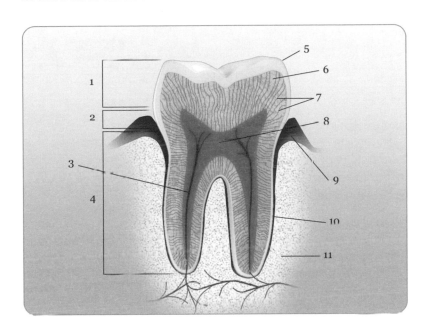

1. _____

2. _____

3. _____

4. _____

5. _____

6. _____

7. _____

8. _____

9. _____

10. _____

11. _____

root canal
gingiva
crown
dentin
cementum
pulp cavity
enamel
bone
dentin tubules
root
neck

Alimentary Canal

The main part of the digestive system is the alimentary canal. It is also called the GI tract (gastrointestinal tract). This is a generic term given for the tube that extends from the lips to the anus. It is coiled, varies in diameter, and the parts are identified individually. However, it never branches and is, in fact, a single continuous tube. The alimentary canal is approximately nine meters (or 30 feet) long and is made up of four layers of tunica (coat or covering).

- Serosa
- Muscularis, consisting of the inner and outer muscularis
- Submucosa
- Mucosa

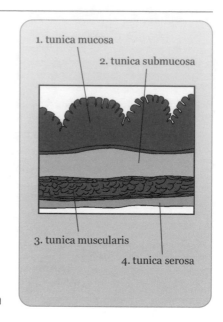

1. tunica mucosa
2. tunica submucosa
3. tunica muscularis
4. tunica serosa

Tunica serosa

This is the outermost covering of the alimentary canal. In most of the digestive tract (stomach and intestines), it consists of a thin layer of loose connective tissue covered by mesothelium (a type of squamous epithelium [single layer of skin cells] that lines body cavities within the peritoneal cavity). This structure is also referred to as visceral peritoneum, as it covers all of the vital organs.

In the abdominal cavity, the serosa on each side of the lumen (tube) fuses together to form a suspensory structure called mesentery. This structure houses blood vessels and nerves that supply the digestive tract and is continuous for the length of the cavity lining. Outside of the abdominal cavity, the digestive lumen connects to such structures as the esophagus and rectum by way of a layer of connective tissue called the tunica adventitia.

Tunica muscularis (inner and outer)

This gives the alimentary canal the ability to be motile (having the ability of spontaneous movement). In most of the alimentary canal, muscularis consists of two thick layers (inner and outer muscularis) of smooth muscle (involuntary muscles with a single nuclei, spindle-like in appearance). The muscle fibers of the inner layer are aligned circularly, whereas those in the outer layer are aligned longitudinally. This combination of circular and longitudinal smooth muscle gives the tube an ability to perform complex movements that squeeze and propel solid or liquid nutrients in the lumen (a process called peristalsis). Additionally, the muscularis contains valves or sphincters. These are especially thickened circular muscles that occur in strategic places within the canal to regulate food passage. Between the inner circular and outer longitudinal layers of smooth muscle is another critical component of the digestive tract's nervous system—the myenteric (muscle + intestine) plexus.

Tunica submucosa

This layer lies between the mucosal and inner muscularis layers. This layer is highly vascular (containing many blood vessels). It is composed of elastic and collagen fibers, and its function is to serve the mucosal layer. The submucosa also contains the submucous plexus, a critical component of the digestive tract's nervous system that provides nervous control to the mucosa.

Tunica mucosa

This is the innermost layer of the alimentary canal that lines the digestive tract. Of the four tunic layers, the mucosa is the most widely varied. It allows the lumen the ability to perform digestive tasks along its length. Included within the tunica mucosa are epithelium cells vital to the functions of absorption and more. Beneath the epithelium, but still within the tunica mucosa, is a layer called the lamina propria, which is loose connective tissue. Blood vessels and lymphatics course through the lamina propria to supply the epithelium.

Beneath the lamina propria is the lamina muscularis mucosae, a thin layer of smooth muscle that allows the mucosa to move and fold.

Three primary functions of this layer are:

Distention: the state of being enlarged or allowing for an increased capacity. This occurs most notably in the stomach.

Absorption: the process of absorbing or assimilating nutrients, such as in the small intestine, or the absorption of water in the colon.

Secretion: where the glandular parts secrete digestive enzymes into the cavity to break down food, such as in the stomach.

I. **FILL IN THE BLANK.**
   Enter the bolded terms in the space provided.

   1. **tunica mucosa** _____

   2. **tunica muscularis** _____

   3. **tunica serosa** _____

   4. **tunica submucosa** _____

II. FILL IN THE BLANK.

Refer to the image and enter the term corresponding to the following numbers. Use the words in the box to fill in the blanks.

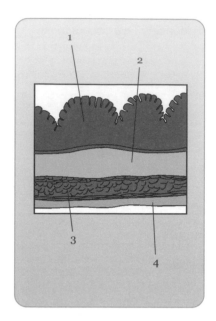

1. _____

2. _____

3. _____

4. _____

tunica muscularis
tunica mucosa
tunica serosa
tunica submucosa

Structures of the Alimentary Canal

As you are exposed to the examination, diagnosis, and treatment of gastrointestinal disorders in individual reports, the term "alimentary canal" or even "gastrointestinal tract" are far too general to be practical from a medical perspective, and thus you will rarely see them in transcribed reports. The same is true of larger components of the GI tract. The large intestine is a familiar term to many people from basic biology in high school or college; however, in a medical context this term is too general to be useful. It is necessary for medical practitioners to determine a specific component of the large intestine, such as the sigmoid colon or hepatic flexure, where a problem may exist. It is these individual parts of the tract that are identified on x-rays, CT scans, or in operative procedures.

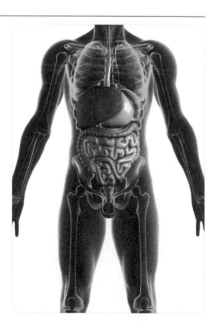

In addition to the individual organs that make up the digestive system, there are many microscopic glandular structures that are found in the walls of the GI tract.

There are also larger secretory organs (such as the liver and pancreas) whose products are transmitted through ducts within the GI tract. These secretions break fats into fatty acids, proteins into amino acids, and carbohydrates into simple sugars. Only after food is broken down is it able to be used by the body for nutrition.

Essentially, the greater part of the gastrointestinal tract itself is contained within the abdominal cavity. The abdominal cavity is lined by the parietal peritoneum. On the back (or the dorsal side) the peritoneum itself forms long, thin sheets of tissue that support the GI tract. This is called the dorsal mesentery. Each organ or structure within the abdominal cavity also has its own protective lining called visceral peritoneum or serosa.

Where two organs are next to each other, double folds of peritoneum called omentum pass between them to support and transmit vessels and nerves to and from the organs. This omentum also protects the organs from excessive rubbing that would break down outer organ walls.

The omentum is divided into two sections:

1. **lesser omentum**. The lesser omentum extends from the lesser curvature of the stomach to the underside of the liver.
2. **greater omentum**. The greater omentum extends from the greater curvature of the stomach to the transverse colon.

There are some abdominal organs positioned outside the peritoneal cavity, meaning they are not covered by peritoneum. These are referred to as retroperitoneal and include the pancreas, kidneys, most of the duodenum, and the abdominal aorta.

If you think about it, you already know a great deal about the process of digestion. For example, you take food into your mouth (also called the oral or buccal cavity). You taste it, chew it, and swallow it. The mouth and its components (e.g , lips, teeth, tongue) are vital to the process of digestion. The terms for these particular structures are part of our everyday vernacular, so they will not be further discussed in this chapter. However, there are, of course, medical designations for the same terms.

A lip is a labium (plural: labia), and lingual means "pertaining to the tongue." The tongue is connected to the floor of the mouth by the lingual frenulum. You know that lingua refers to the tongue, and a frenulum is a general term for a membrane that curbs or limits the movement of an organ or part. Finally, the tongue has many small elevations on it that are called papillae. These are also important in the process of digestion.

That specialty of medicine that deals specifically with digestion and problems associated with it is gastroenterology. In a hospital setting, gastroenterology is part of the medical record and will be integrated together with many other specialties. Consider 30 feet of digestive tract, and you can imagine the numerous problems that can occur.

Additionally, factor in how important the intake of food or nutrition is to sustaining life. Illnesses related to digestion and nutrition and the treatment of such illnesses is a major part of medicine. It will be necessary for you to be familiar with the anatomical and disease terms found in this unit.

I. MULTIPLE CHOICE.
Choose the best answer.

1. The lining of the abdominal cavity.

   ○ parietal perineum

   ○ omentum

   ○ viscera

   ○ parietal peritoneum

2. The branch of medicine dealing with digestion.

   ○ genitourinary

   ○ gastroenterology

   ○ gastrologist

   ○ gerentologist

3. The outer and final layer of the GI tract.

   ○ omentum

   ○ serosa

   ○ adventitia

   ○ retroperitoneal

4. The process of assimilating nutrients.

   ○ gastroenterology

   ○ absorption

   ○ distention

   ○ secretion

5. Double folds of peritoneum.

   ○ serosa

   ○ omentum

   ○ peritoneum

   ○ adventitia

6. A term for releasing enzymes to break down food.

   ○ secretion

   ○ secretive

   ○ distending

   ○ peristalsis

7. Another term for visceral peritoneum.
   - ⃝ submucosa
   - ⃝ serosa
   - ⃝ mucosa
   - ⃝ adventitia

8. The canal which makes up most of the digestive system.
   - ⃝ digestive canal
   - ⃝ alimentary canal
   - ⃝ gastroenterology canal
   - ⃝ absorptive canal

9. The layer responsible for contraction.
   - ⃝ muscularis
   - ⃝ collagen
   - ⃝ lumen
   - ⃝ serosa

10. Organs not covered by the peritoneum.
    - ⃝ peritoneal
    - ⃝ viscera
    - ⃝ retroperitoneal
    - ⃝ submucosa

11. Long, thin sheets of tissue that support the GI tract.
    - ⃝ serosa
    - ⃝ lumen
    - ⃝ dorsal mesentery
    - ⃝ peritoneum

12. The approximate length of the GI tract.
    - ⃝ 40 feet
    - ⃝ 25 feet
    - ⃝ 30 feet
    - ⃝ 13 feet

13. The second layer surrounding the lumen.
    - ⃝ serosa
    - ⃝ submucosa
    - ⃝ viscera
    - ⃝ omentum

14. The state of being enlarged.

- ○ distention
- ○ retention
- ○ absorption
- ○ intention

15. Along with elastic fibers, this comprises the submucosal layer.

- ○ papillae
- ○ serosa
- ○ muscularis
- ○ collagen

16. The process of moving through the tract.

- ○ swallowing
- ○ peristalsis
- ○ secretion
- ○ absorption

17. The liver and pancreas are _____ organs.

- ○ inguinal
- ○ absorptive
- ○ secretory
- ○ mucosal

18. Extending from the larger curvature of the stomach to the transverse colon.

- ○ adventitia
- ○ greater omentum
- ○ parietal peritoneum
- ○ lesser omentum

19. Not a function of digestion.

- ○ absorption
- ○ secretion
- ○ distention
- ○ support

Review: Upper Digestive Structures

I. SPELLING.
Determine if the following words are spelled correctly. If the spelling is correct, leave the word as it has already been entered. If the spelling is incorrect, provide the correct spelling.

1. papilae _____

2. gastrointerology _____

3. distension _____

4. lingual _____

5. peritoneum _____

6. mucosa _____

7. mesentary _____

8. omentum _____

9. lumen _____

10. paristalsis _____

II. MATCHING.
Match the correct term to the definition. Enter only the letter in the space provided (no punctuation).

1. ____ The outer layer of the alimentary canal.

2. ____ Double folds of peritoneum.

3. ____ The hollow part of a tube or tubular organ.

4. ____ Organs not covered by the peritoneum.

5. ____ Another name for the mouth.

6. ____ Describes the body from the chest to the hips.

7. ____ Extends from the larger curvature of the stomach to the transverse colon.

8. ____ Refers to the GI tract of an embryo.

9. ____ Means pertaining to the tongue.

10. ____ Term which means literally "pertaining to the cheek."

A. oral cavity
B. omentum
C. gut
D. lumen
E. greater omentum
F. abdomen
G. tunica adventitia
H. buccal
I. lingual
J. retroperitoneal

III. **MULTIPLE CHOICE.**
Choose the best answer.

1. The branch of medicine dealing with digestion.
   ○ gastrenterology
   ○ gastroenterology
   ○ gastronterology
   ○ gastric enterology

2. The lining of the coelomic cavity.
   ○ parietal perineum
   ○ parietal peroneum
   ○ parental peritoneum
   ○ parietal peritoneum

3. Elevations on the tongue.
   ○ papillae
   ○ papilla
   ○ papilae
   ○ parpellae

4. Another name for organs.
   ○ viscera
   ○ visera
   ○ vicera
   ○ vissera

5. The process of assimilating nutrients.
   ○ absarption
   ○ absorption
   ○ absorpsion
   ○ absorptive

6. The tongue is connected to the floor of the mouth via the _____.
   ○ lingual frenulum
   ○ lingual phrenulum
   ○ lingual frenulem
   ○ lingual phrenulem

7. Along with elastic fibers, this comprises the submucosal layer.
   - ○ colagen
   - ○ collajen
   - ○ colagin
   - ○ collagen

8. The process of moving through the tract.
   - ○ parastalsis
   - ○ peristalsis
   - ○ paristalsis
   - ○ peristolsis

9. The approximate length of the GI tract.
   - ○ 30 meters
   - ○ 30 inches
   - ○ 30 feet
   - ○ 3 feet

10. Not a function of digestion.
    - ○ absorption
    - ○ secretion
    - ○ distention
    - ○ support

Major Structures of the Digestive System

The following are figures of the major structures of the digestive system. Note the placement of the individual components of the alimentary canal.

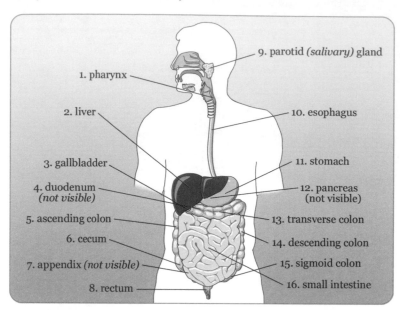

9. parotid *(salivary)* gland
1. pharynx
2. liver
3. gallbladder
4. duodenum *(not visible)*
5. ascending colon
6. cecum
7. appendix *(not visible)*
8. rectum
10. esophagus
11. stomach
12. pancreas *(not visible)*
13. transverse colon
14. descending colon
15. sigmoid colon
16. small intestine

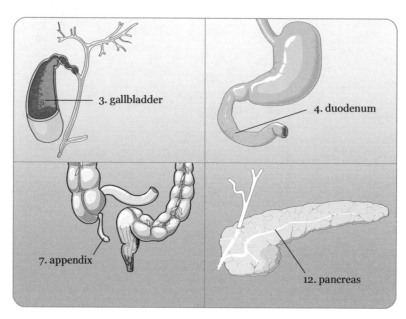

3. gallbladder
4. duodenum
7. appendix
12. pancreas

I. FILL IN THE BLANK.
Enter the bolded terms in the space provided.

1. **appendix** _____

2. **ascending colon** _____

3. **cecum** _____

4. **descending colon** _____

5. **duodenum** _____

6. **esophagus** _____

7. **gallbladder** _____

8. **liver** _____

9. **pancreas** _____

10. **parotid (salivary) gland** _____

11. **pharynx** _____

12. **rectum** _____

13. **sigmoid colon** _____

14. **small intestine** _____

15. **stomach** _____

16. **transverse colon** _____

II. FILL IN THE BLANK.
Please enter the numbered terms in the blanks provided. Use the word(s) in the box to fill in the blanks.

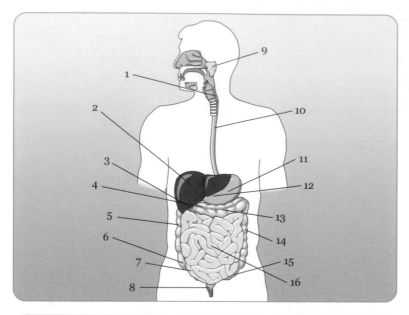

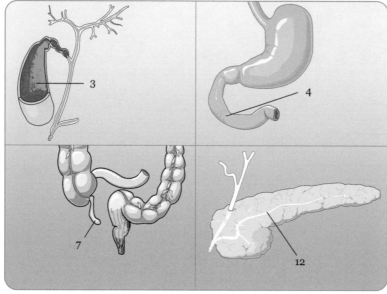

1. _____

2. _____

3. _____

4. _____

5. _____

6. _____

7. _____

8. _____

9. _____

10. _____

11. _____

12. _____

13. _____

14. _____

15. _____

16. _____

parotid (salivary) gland
small intestine
duodenum
transverse colon
gallbladder
sigmoid colon
ascending colon
descending colon
appendix
esophagus
pharynx
pancreas
rectum
liver
stomach
cecum

Mouth and Esophagus

Before continuing, it may be easier for you to learn additional terms if you are better acquainted with their nature and function.

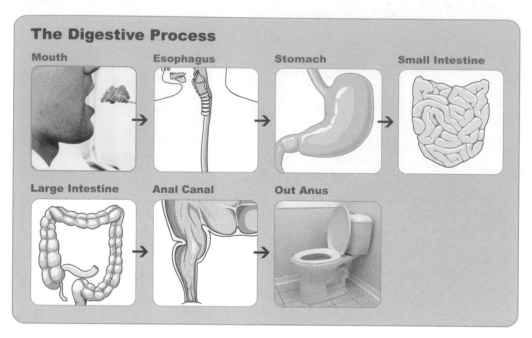

Mouth, Esophagus, Stomach

Common sense dictates that your mouth is where you put your food. This is the very beginning of the digestive process.

Next, you use your teeth to chew food or break it down into smaller particles that are easier for your body to process. To move on to the next phase, you swallow. At this point food enters the pharynx, which serves as a common passageway for both the respiratory system (which will be discussed in greater detail soon) and the digestive system.

There are separate components of the pharynx. The nasopharynx is a posterior continuation of the nasal cavity and is not actually part of the digestive system. The uvula is a small, fleshy mass that hangs from the soft palate, just above the base of the tongue. The oropharynx is a combination of the roots oro- (meaning relationship to the mouth) and pharynx, and extends from the soft palate within the mouth to the level of the hyoid bone. Also in this region is the epiglottis, which is a lid-like structure composed of cartilage that hangs over the entrance to the larynx to prevent food from entering the larynx or trachea upon swallowing.

The esophagus is the part of the alimentary canal that connects the pharynx to the stomach. It is a muscular tube that is about 25 cm long. The muscular function of the esophagus is not voluntary, but carries food quickly from one place to another.

There are eight steps that occur to get food from the mouth to the stomach:

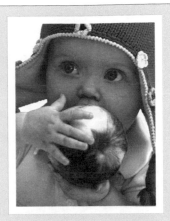

1. The food is chewed up and moistened with saliva to become a bolus, or a rounded mass of food.
2. The bolus is pushed to the back of the mouth by the tongue and the cheeks.
3. The soft palate and pendant uvula seal off the nasal cavity.
4. The tip of the tongue pushes up against the top of the mouth while the base of the tongue pushes the food down, and the sides of the pharynx contract.
5. The hyoid bone and the larynx are elevated.
6. The bolus pushes down on the epiglottis, which blocks the trachea.
7. A contraction of the pharynx pushes the bolus into the esophagus, past the larynx.
8. Another wave of contractions pushes the bolus through the esophagus to the stomach. The muscles of the neck and throat then relax and return to their normal breathing position.

I. **MATCHING.**
Match the correct term to the definition.

1. ____ pharynx
2. ____ uvula
3. ____ oropharynx
4. ____ epiglottis
5. ____ esophagus

A. small, fleshy mass hanging from the soft palate
B. lid-like structure that hangs over the entrance to the larynx
C. extends from the soft palate in the mouth to the level of the hyoid bone
D. part of the alimentary canal that connects the pharynx to the stomach
E. passageway for the respiratory and digestive system

Stomach

The stomach is the most distended portion of the alimentary canal. It serves primarily as storage for food before it passes into the intestines. Although some digestion occurs at this point, food is primarily only converted into a pasty material.

The stomach consists of four major parts:

1. **Cardiac orifice** is the junction between the esophagus and the stomach. This is also frequently referred to as the *GE junction* (gastroesophageal junction). Although no true sphincter exists at this point, the muscles here are in a constant state of contraction in order to prevent the stomach contents from flowing backward.
2. The **fundus** is the dome-shaped portion of the stomach that extends slightly above the cardiac orifice.
3. The **body** of the stomach is the widest portion and is located between the lesser and greater curvatures.
4. The **pylorus** of the stomach is the last area of the stomach, just before the duodenum.

I. TRUE/FALSE.
Mark the following true or false.

1. Food is mostly digested in the stomach, before it passes into the intestines.

   ○ true
   ○ false

2. The fundus is the last area of the stomach, just before the duodenum

   ○ true
   ○ false

3. The muscles in the cardiac orifice are constantly contracted to prevent the contents of the stomach from flowing backward.

   ○ true
   ○ false

4. The pylorus is a dome-shaped portion of the stomach.

   ○ true
   ○ false

5. The widest portion of the stomach between the lesser and greater curvatures is called the body of the stomach.

   ○ true
   ○ false

Small Intestine and Large Intestine

After the food bolus leaves the stomach it enters the small intestine. This is actually the longest portion of the alimentary canal. It measures approximately 21 feet long and is 2.5 cm wide. It is called the "small intestine" because it is smaller in diameter than the next portion of the alimentary canal. The small intestine is divided into the following three main regions:

- duodenum (This receives secretions from the liver and the pancreas)
- jejunum
- ileum (The small intestine makes the transition to the large intestine here through what is called the ileocecal valve)

Highlights

The large intestine, where most water is absorbed and feces are formed, consists of four major regions:

1. cecum
2. colon
3. rectum
4. anus/anal canal

The distal-most portion of the alimentary canal is the large intestine. It is so named because at 6 cm in diameter, it is the widest portion of the canal. It is here that most water is absorbed and feces are formed.

It is divided into four major regions:

Cecum

The cecum opens into the colon and has the appendix, a small finger-like projection that is attached to its medial portion.

Colon

The second portion of the large intestine is the colon. Different areas of the colon have specific terms assigned to them. At approximately the liver, the colon bends sharply, and this area is referred to as the hepatic flexure. The colon then extends in a horizontal direction, and that portion is called the transverse colon. At the left abdominal wall, there is another sharp bend in the colon. This is called the splenic flexure and is the beginning of the descending colon, or that portion of the large intestine that goes downward (descends). Finally, the colon terminates in an S-shaped bend that is referred to as the sigmoid colon.

Rectum

Next is the rectum, which is a tube approximately 15 cm long located between the sigmoid colon and the anal canal.

Anus/Anal Canal

The anal canal forms a muscular opening in the muscles of the pelvic floor that is called the anus. This is surrounded by both involuntary and voluntary muscular sphincters.

I. **TRUE/FALSE.**
Mark the following true or false.

1. The large intestine is the longest portion of the alimentary canal

   ○ true
   ○ false

2. The duodenum, in the small Intestine, receives secretions from the liver and pancreas.

   ○ true
   ○ false

3. The small intestine transitions to the large intestine at the ileum

   ○ true
   ○ false

II. **FILL IN THE BLANK.**
Using the word/word parts in the box, fill in the blanks.

1. The s-shaped bend where the colon ends is called the

   _____.

2. The _____ opens into the colon and contains the appendix.

3. The area near the liver where the colon bends sharply is referred to as the _____.

splenic flexure
rectum
cecum
hepatic flexure
sigmoid colon
anal canal

4. The _____ is the beginning of the descending
    colon.

5. The _____ forms a muscular opening in the anus.

6. The tube between the sigmoid colon and anal canal is called the

    _____ .

Large Organs of the Digestive System

The large intestine has a larger diameter than the small intestine. There are other differences as well. There are no villi in the large intestine. There are three distinct longitudinal muscles, teniae coli, which run the length of the large intestine. There is also a series of bulges in the wall of the large intestine that are called sacculations or haustra.

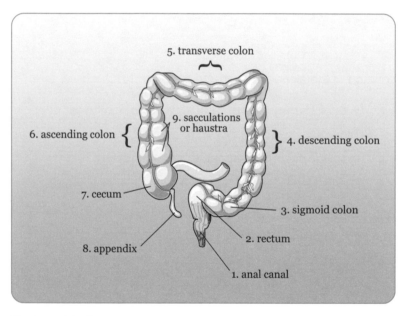

The Large Intestines

Although the alimentary canal comprises most of the digestive system, there are a few accessory organs that secrete directly into the alimentary canal via ducts, and these are important to digestion. They include the liver, the gallbladder, and the pancreas.

Liver

The liver is the largest gland in the body. It is made up of many liver lobules that produce bile. Bile is continuously secreted into the intestines and is very important to digestion.

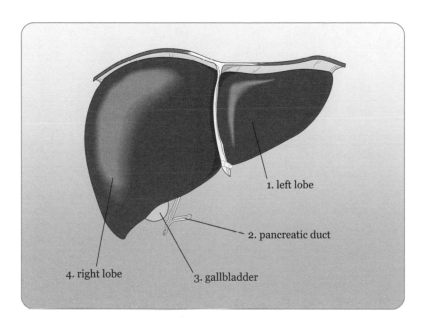

1. left lobe

2. pancreatic duct

4. right lobe

3. gallbladder

Gallbladder

The gallbladder is a sac-like organ that is attached to the undersurface of the liver. It stores and concentrates bile. The cystic duct drains the gallbladder. It unites with the hepatic duct to form the common bile duct that conveys bile into the duodenum.

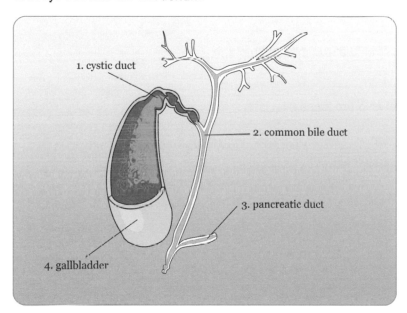

1. cystic duct

2. common bile duct

3. pancreatic duct

4. gallbladder

Pancreas

Finally, the pancreas is involved in both the digestive and the endocrine systems. For its role in digestion, it creates juices and secretes them into the duodenum for the breakdown of foods.

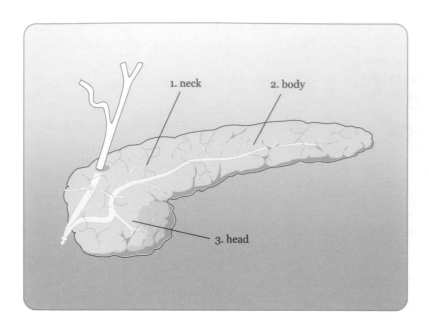

1. neck   2. body

3. head

I. FILL IN THE BLANK.
Using the word/word parts in the box, fill in the blanks.

1. The organ that creates and secretes juices into the duodenum for breakdown of foods is the _____.

2. The three distinct longitudinal muscles that run the length of the large intestine are called _____.

3. The largest gland in the body, that also produces bile, is the _____.

4. The organ that stores and concentrates bile is the _____.

| liver |
| teniae coli |
| gallbladder |
| pancreas |

II. FILL IN BLANK.

In the blanks provided below, refer to the above image and enter the term corresponding to the following numbers. Use the word(s) in the box to fill in the blanks.

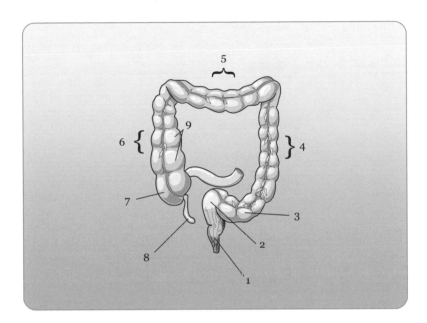

1. _____

2. _____

3. _____

4. _____

5. _____

6. _____

7. _____

8. _____

9. _____

transverse colon
anal canal
appendix
sacculations or haustra
sigmoid colon
ascending colon
rectum
descending colon
cecum

Review: Digestive Structures

I. FILL IN THE BLANK.
   Enter the bolded terms in the space provided.

1. **nasopharynx** _____   2. **uvula** _____

3. **palate** _____   4. **oropharynx** _____

5. **epiglottis** _____   6. **esophagus** _____

7. **bolus** _____   8. **stomach** _____

9. **cardiac orifice** _____   10. **fundus** _____

11. **body** _____   12. **pylorus** _____

13. **duodenum** _____   14. **jejunum** _____

15. **ileum** _____   16. **ileocecal valve** _____

17. **cecum** _____   18. **colon** _____

19. **rectum** _____   20. **appendix** _____

21. **ascending colon** _____   22. **hepatic flexure** _____

23. **transverse colon** _____   24. **splenic flexure** _____

25. **descending colon** _____   26. **sigmoid colon** _____

27. **anal canal** _____   28. **anus** _____

29. **sphincters** _____   30. **villi** _____

31. **teniae coli** _____   32. **sacculations** _____

33. **haustra** _____   34. **cystic duct** _____

35. **hepatic duct** _____   36. **common bile duct** _____

37. **GE junction** _____

II. MULTIPLE CHOICE.
Choose the best answer.

1. Which of the following is not an accessory organ?
   ○ splenic flexure
   ○ liver
   ○ pancreas
   ○ gallbladder

2. Bulges in the large intestinal wall.
   ○ hernias
   ○ sacculations
   ○ fasciculations
   ○ occlusions

3. A rounded mass of food.
   ○ ball
   ○ dome
   ○ fundus
   ○ bolus

4. Dome shaped portion of the stomach.
   ○ fundus
   ○ bolus
   ○ gut
   ○ abdomen

5. A small, fleshy mass above the tongue.
   ○ palate
   ○ adenoid
   ○ uvula
   ○ frenulum

6. Part of the small intestine that receives secretions from the liver and pancreas
   ○ splenic flexure
   ○ duodenum
   ○ spleen
   ○ fundus

7. Where small and large intestines meet.

○ iliocecal valve
○ splenic flexure
○ cecum
○ ileocecal valve

8. Bend in the colon, left of the abdomen.

○ duodenum
○ splenic flexure
○ ileocecal valve
○ stomach

9. 15-cm portion of the large intestine.

○ rectum
○ cecum
○ small intestine
○ esophagus

10. Finger-like structure off the cecum.

○ spleen
○ uvula
○ rectum
○ appendix

11. Cartilage that hangs over the larynx.

○ epiglottis
○ uvula
○ tonsil
○ frenulum

12. The most distended portion of the alimentary canal.

○ abdomen
○ stomach
○ bolus
○ duodenum

13. Between the pharynx and the stomach.

    ○ uvula
    ○ cecum
    ○ esophagus
    ○ appendix

14. The first part of the large intestine.

    ○ cecum
    ○ small intestine
    ○ duodenum
    ○ rectum

III. **FILL IN THE BLANK.**
    Use the word(s) in the box to fill in the blanks.

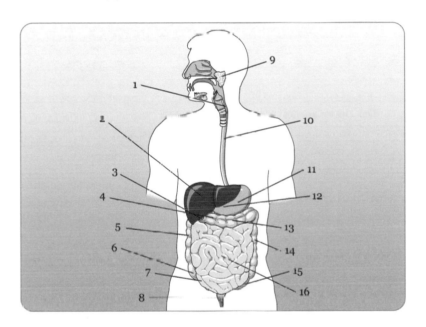

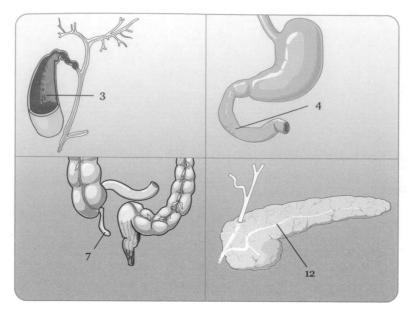

1. _____
2. _____
3. _____
4. _____
5. _____
6. _____
7. _____
8. _____
9. _____
10. _____
11. _____
12. _____
13. _____
14. _____
15. _____
16. _____

transverse colon

gallbladder

small intestine

duodenum

pancreas

ascending colon

parotid (salivary) gland

descending colon

pharynx

appendix

esophagus

sigmoid colon

liver

stomach

cecum

rectum

Disease Processes

Try for a moment to imagine the vast array of consumable (and nonconsumable) materials that can be taken into one's body via the gastrointestinal system. If you draw upon personal experience, you can probably remember something you ate that "didn't agree with you," or perhaps, that carried a nasty parasite.

The GI system is one system over which individuals have a great deal of control. Consequently, many of the problems associated with it are related to what goes (or does not go) into our mouths. Factors that directly affect digestive system performance range from too little water (dehydration), to insufficient nutrients (malnutrition), to spices and fat we voluntarily add, to bacteria and parasites that we inadvertently consume. The quality and quantity of fluids and nutrients we take in can greatly impact our gastrointestinal health.

Furthermore, the scope of potential problems is, to say the least, broad. In diagnosing gastrointestinal problems, there are relatively few symptoms that alert healthcare professionals to the nature of a GI problem. Unless you are extraordinarily lucky, most of them should be familiar to you from personal experience. As you encounter terminology exercises, rewrite the term in the blank and take time to read and correlate the definition to the term.

Symptoms of Gastrointestinal Illness

The following symptoms are all indicative of some underlying gastrointestinal pathology. They can be determined either subjectively (by taking a patient history) or through observation by a healthcare professional in a physical examination (during which symptoms can be observed and tenderness, redness, swelling, bloating, or other symptoms determined).

In addition to a consideration of the symptoms exhibited by a patient, the etiology of gastrointestinal problems can be determined by means of several different types of tests. For example, many nutrients should be present in specific quantities in the blood, and these can be studied through laboratory workups. Other bodily fluids can also be examined by the laboratory (throat culture, urine, and stool, to name a few). Physicians also palpate certain areas of the throat or abdomen or observe conditions in the throat or over the skin with various noninvasive instruments.

I. **TERMINOLOGY.**
   Enter each term in the space provided. Read the definition and description for each term.

   1. **anorexia** _____

   A loss or total lack of appetite.

   2. **borborygmi** _____

   The audible rumbling sounds of gas moving through the intestinal tract. This is the plural form. The singular form is borborygmus or borborygmos.

   3. **chills** _____

   A shivering or a shaking.

   4. **rigor** _____

   Shivering or trembling, usually accompanied by fever; also called chills.

5. **constipation** _____

Infrequent or difficult evacuation of feces. This term could be classified as either a symptom or a disease. Patients can subjectively relate that they are experiencing the discomfort of constipation, and it can also be the diagnosis.

6. **obstipation** _____

Constipation that continues for a prolonged period of time.

7. **dysphagia** _____

This is a subjective feeling of difficulty swallowing. It occurs when there is impaired progression of the food bolus from the pharynx to the stomach.

8. **fever** _____

An elevation in temperature above normal. This is also called pyrexia. If a patient has a fever, physicians will usually refer to that patient as being febrile.

9. **afebrile** _____

Not having a fever.

10. **flatus** _____

Gas produced by bacterial action on waste matter in the intestines. Composed primarily of hydrogen sulfide and methane.

11. **bloating** _____

The feeling of excessive gas in the colon.

12. **belching** _____

Expressing of excessive gas through the mouth.

13. **flatulence** _____

Expressing of excessive gas through the anus.

14. **heartburn** _____

A retrosternal sensation of burning felt in waves and arising upward toward the neck.

15. **hematemesis** _____
Vomiting of blood.

16. **hematochezia** _____

The passage of bloody stools.

17. **melena** _____

Melan(o)- is a combining form that means black. The term melena refers both to the passage of dark and pithy stools stained with blood pigment, and black vomit. Although the combining form is spelled with an A, it is important to note that the term melena or melenic stools is spelled with an E.

18. **nausea** _____

An unpleasant sensation in the epigastric and abdominal area, which often results in vomiting.

19. **odynophagia** _____

Pain during swallowing.

20. **pallor** _____

Paleness or the absence of skin color.

21. **regurgitation** _____

Flow in the opposite direction than is normal.

22. **tenesmus** _____

Straining, especially ineffective and painful straining during a bowel movement or urination.

23. **vomiting** _____

Also called emesis. The forcible expulsion of stomach contents through the mouth. (Try not to think about it.)

24. **weakness** _____

Lacking physical strength.

25. **weight loss** _____

This is self-explanatory: losing pounds.

II. **MULTIPLE CHOICE.**
   Choose the best answer.

   1. Painful straining with urination or defecation.

      ○ spasm
      ○ melena
      ○ dysphagia
      ○ tenesmus

   2. Normal temperature.

      ○ afebrile
      ○ febrile
      ○ clammy
      ○ 98.5

   3. Flow in an opposite direction than is normal.

      ○ diarrhea
      ○ regurgitation
      ○ constipation
      ○ digestion

4. Bulges in the wall of the large intestine.
   ○ haustra
   ○ hernia
   ○ obstruction
   ○ bolus

5. A ring-like band of muscle fibers which constricts a passage or closes an orifice.
   ○ fundus
   ○ sphincter
   ○ spleen
   ○ alimentary canal

6. Infrequent or difficult passage of stool.
   ○ diarrhea
   ○ melena
   ○ constipation
   ○ hematochezia

7. A burning felt in the epigastrium, moving in waves towards the neck.
   ○ heartburn
   ○ febrile
   ○ afebrile
   ○ gas

8. A rounded mass of food.
   ○ haustra
   ○ blockage
   ○ bolus
   ○ obstruction

9. Rumblies in the tumbly.
   ○ hunger pains
   ○ borborygmi
   ○ gas
   ○ flatulence

10. The absence of skin pigment.
    ○ white
    ○ melena
    ○ pallor
    ○ fever

11. Lacking physical strength.

   ○ amuscular
   ○ muscular
   ○ weakness
   ○ strength

12. Expulsion of excessive gas from the colon.

   ○ flatulence
   ○ dysphagia
   ○ constipation
   ○ diarrhea

13. Lack of appetite.

   ○ diet
   ○ nausea
   ○ anorexia
   ○ heartburn

14. The passage of bloody stools.

   ○ melena
   ○ hematemesis
   ○ obstipation
   ○ hematochezia

15. Pyrexia, or an elevation of normal body temperature.

   ○ febrile
   ○ afebrile
   ○ chills
   ○ rigors

16. Painful swallowing.

   ○ dysphagia
   ○ dysphasia
   ○ odynophagia
   ○ obstipation

17. The passage of black, tarry stools.

   ○ melena
   ○ hematochezia
   ○ diarrhea
   ○ hematemesis

18. Vomiting blood.

○ vomiting
○ hematemesis
○ hemtochezia
○ obstipation

19. An unpleasant sensation in the stomach, which often leads to vomiting.

○ heartburn
○ gas
○ nausea
○ flatulence

20. Forcible expulsion of stomach contents through the mouth.

○ vomiting
○ obstipation
○ odynophagia
○ dysphagia

21. Intractable constipation.

○ tenesmus
○ hematochezia
○ melena
○ obstipation

22. Difficulty in swallowing.

○ dysphasia
○ odynophagia
○ dysphagia
○ regurgitation

Gastrointestinal Disorders – Lesson 1

Other symptoms, malformations, and abnormalities are also indicative of gastrointestinal disorders. However, the ones listed here are by far the most common. There is a wide array of possible maladies that are determinable based upon these common symptoms, their frequency, intensity, and the unique combination of manifestations.

In addition to abnormal values found in the blood, there are viral, bacterial, and parasite components that primarily affect the GI system. As mentioned previously, the food and drink that we choose to put in (or not put in) our bodies greatly impacts the health of the alimentary canal and are catalysts for many of these diseases.

In the following lists, enter the indicated term and read their descriptions. These are all fairly common problems associated with the digestive system and are often seen in hospital and clinic health care reports.

I. TERMINOLOGY.
Enter each term in the space provided. Read the definition and description for each term.

1. achalasia _____

This is an impairment of normal esophageal peristalsis. (You may remember that peristalsis is the movement of the muscles in the alimentary canal to propel the food bolus.) It also affects the ability of the lower esophageal sphincter to relax. The most common symptoms are dysphagia, regurgitation, nocturnal cough, and chest pain.

2. anorexia nervosa _____

This is a mental condition characterized by an individual's refusal to eat enough to maintain a minimal body weight, usually fueled by an intense fear of becoming obese.

3. appendicitis _____

Inflammation of the vermiform appendix. (The term *appendix* is actually a general term which means a supplementary, accessory, or dependent part of a main structure.) This is the first, but many individual structures which are found in the body (GI system and elsewhere) can be individually affected by infection which causes inflammation. You will notice that the suffix -itis appears in several disease processes.

4. vermiform _____

The vermiform appendix specifically identifies the diverticulum of the cecum. However, healthcare professionals commonly drop the term *vermiform* when referring to this particular appendix.

5. atresia _____

The absence or closure of a normal body orifice or tubular organ.

6. bezoar _____

Tightly packed, partially digested agglomerations of hair or vegetable matter. Seeds, bubble gum, medication, and other materials can mimic true bezoars.

7. botulism _____

A type of food poisoning caused by the production of the bacteria Clostridium botulinum in improperly canned foods. It is characterized by vomiting, abdominal pain, difficulty seeing, dryness of the mouth and pharynx, dyspepsia, cough; it often results in death.

8. cheiloschisis _____

This is another term for cleft lip or harelip. It is a congenital abnormality.

9. cholecystitis _____

Inflammation of the gallbladder. There are different types of cholecystitis, the most common being chronic and acute. An acute infection generally indicates severe infection and often necessitates a cholecystectomy, which is removal of the gallbladder. This is an extremely common procedure.

10. cholelithiasis _____

The presence or formation of gallstones.

II. SPELLING.

Determine if the following words are spelled correctly. If the spelling is correct, leave the word as it has already been entered. If the spelling is incorrect, provide the correct spelling.

1. cholecystitis _____

2. verniform _____

3. chelioschisis _____

4. anorexia nerosa _____

5. appendecitis _____

III. MULTIPLE CHOICE.
Choose the best answer.

1. Impairment of normal esophageal peristalsis.
   - ○ akalasia
   - ○ achalasia
   - ○ acalasia
   - ○ achalazia

2. Tightly packed, partially digested ball of hair.
   - ○ bizoar
   - ○ bezoar
   - ○ bezaor
   - ○ bizaor

3. Type of food poisoning caused by improperly canned foods.
   - ○ botulism
   - ○ bochulism
   - ○ bochulysm
   - ○ botulysm

4. The absence or closure of a normal body opening.
   - ○ atrisia
   - ○ atrisea
   - ○ atressia
   - ○ atresia

5. The presence or formation of gallstones.
   - ○ cholelithiasis
   - ○ chololethiasis
   - ○ cholelethiasis
   - ○ choleithiasis

Gastrointestinal Disorders – Lesson 2

I. TERMINOLOGY.
Enter each term in the space provided. Read the definition and description for each term.

1. **cirrhosis** _____

This refers to a group of liver diseases in which the normal hepatic structure is destroyed over time by nodules. It is the third leading cause of death in North America for people 45 to 65 years of age. In North America it is often caused by chronic alcohol abuse. (In other parts of the world it can be caused by untreated and highly communicable strains of hepatitis.)

2. **colitis** _____

Inflammation of the colon.

3. **dehydration** _____

A condition that results from an excessive loss of body water. This can occur on a hot day without a drinking fountain close by, but also occurs when there is vomiting, diarrhea, diabetes, mental disorder, coma, or when a patient is taking diuretic medications (those which promote the excretion of urine). It can be life-threatening.

4. **dental caries** _____

Tooth decay. Although this is a component of the dental specialty, because it directly affects the teeth, which are responsible for masticating food, it is significant to the function of the GI system.

5. **diarrhea** _____

Abnormal frequency and liquidity of fecal discharges. Diarrhea is actually a symptom that suggests the presence of a disorder. However, it often is short in duration, is easily identifiable by a patient, and often does not require any treatment.

6. **diverticulum** _____

An abnormal bulge, pocket, or pouch formed from a hollow or tubular structure.

7. **diverticula** _____

The plural form of diverticulum (The plural of diverticulum is NOT diverticuli; this is a common dictation/transcription error.)

8. **diverticulitis** _____

Inflammation of a diverticulum.

9. **diverticulosis** _____

The presence of diverticula with the absence of diverticulitis, especially in the colon.

10. **Zenker diverticulum** _____

The most common place that a diverticulum occurs is just below the pharynx.

II. MULTIPLE CHOICE.
Choose the best answer.

1. The plural form of diverticulum is (◯diverticulums,◯ diverticula).

2. Tooth decay is also referred to as dental (◯caries,◯ carries).

3. The presence of an abnormal bulge from a tubular structure with the absence of inflammation is (◯diverticulosis,◯ diverticulosous).

4. A (◯Zencker,◯ Zenker) diverticulum is located below the pharynx.

5. The current third leading cause of death is North America is (◯cirrhosis,◯ cirrosis).

III. MATCHING.
Match the correct term to the definition.

1. ____ Inflammation of the colon.

2. ____ The condition which results from an excessive loss of body water.

3. ____ Abnormal frequency and liquidity of fecal discharges.

4. ____ An abnormal bulge, pocket or pouch formed from a hollow or tubular structure.

5. ____ Inflammation of a diverticulum.

A. colitis
B. diverticulum
C. diarrhea
D. dehydration
E. diverticulitis

Gastrointestinal Disorders – Lesson 3

I. TERMINOLOGY.
Enter each term in the space provided. Read the definition and description for each term.

1. **dysentery** _____

Any of a variety of disorders marked by inflammation of the intestines, especially the colon. The symptoms include pain in the abdomen, tenesmus, and frequent stools containing blood and mucus.

2. **amebic dysentery** _____

The most common type of dysentery, due to an ulceration of the bowel caused by amebiasis.

3. **amebiasis** _____

The state of being infected by amebae.

4. **dyspepsia** _____

General term which means impairment to the power or function of digestion. It often refers to discomfort in the epigastric region following a meal, or what many people call "indigestion."

5. **enteritis** _____

Inflammation of the intestine, especially the small intestine. Often this is combined (e.g., enterocolitis).

6. **enterocolitis** _____

Inflammation of both the intestine and colon.

7. **cholera** _____

A form of enteritis that is spread by food and water contaminated with feces. It is much more common in Third World countries.

8. **esophagitis** _____

Inflammation of the esophagus.

9. **fecalith** _____

An intestinal concretion (the process of becoming harder or more solid) formed around a center of fecal matter.

10. **fistula** _____

An abnormal passage or communication between two organs or from an internal organ to the surface of the body. There are several different types. It can occur because of trauma, infection, inflammation, degeneration, necrosis, or other causes.

II. **MULTIPLE CHOICE.**
   Choose the best answer.

   1. An intestinal concretion.
      ○ fecolith
      ○ fecalith
      ○ fecaloth
      ○ flecolith

   2. Disorders marked by inflammation of the intestines, especially the colon.
      ○ disentry
      ○ disentery
      ○ dysentary
      ○ dysentery

3. The state of being infected by amebae.

   ◯ ambiasis
   ◯ amebiasis
   ◯ amebiotic
   ◯ ameboiasis

4. Inflammation of the esophagus.

   ◯ esophagitis
   ◯ esophigitis
   ◯ esophagealitis
   ◯ esophagusitis

5. General term which means impairment to the power or function of digestion.

   ◯ dyspsia
   ◯ dispepsia
   ◯ dypepsia
   ◯ dyspepsia

III. TRUE/FALSE.
Mark the following true or false.

1. Enterocolitis is simply inflammation of the colon.

   ◯ true
   ◯ false

2. Amebic is the most common type of dysentery.

   ◯ true
   ◯ false

3. Cholera is spread by water and food contaminated with feces.

   ◯ true
   ◯ false

4. Enteritis is inflammation of the intestine, especially the large intestine.

   ◯ true
   ◯ false

5. A normal passage or communication between two organs or from an internal organ to the surface of the body is called a fistula.

   ◯ true
   ◯ false

Gastrointestinal Disorders – Lesson 4

I. **TERMINOLOGY.**
   Enter each term in the space provided. Read the definition and description for each term.

1. **gastritis** _____

Inflammation of the stomach. This is commonly combined (e.g., gastroenteritis). This is often a result of a bacteria, and symptoms include anorexia, nausea, diarrhea, abdominal pain, and weakness. Gastritis is also a problem frequently associated with alcohol abuse.

2. **gastroenteritis** _____

Acute inflammation of the lining of the stomach and the intestines.

3. **gastroesophageal reflux disease** _____

The reflux of stomach contents into the esophagus. It is often represented by the acronym GERD (gastroesophageal reflux disease). This is usually caused by an incompetent lower esophageal sphincter. The major symptom is heartburn, although it can lead to several more severe disorders.

4. **halitosis** _____

Offensive breath. This can be real as the result of ingested substances, gingival disease, fermentation of food in the mouth, or associated with systemic diseases such as diabetic acidosis. It can also be imagined and the result of anxiety disorders, obsessive disorders, paranoia, or hypochondria.

5. **hepatitis** _____

Inflammation of the liver. Hepatitis can be due to viral, bacterial, or parasitic factors. They are generally classified by letters (i.e., hepatitis A, hepatitis B, hepatitis C). Some strains are transmitted through feces/oral contact, some through the blood (IV drug use), and some are sexually transmitted. Hepatitis can be chronic and active, in which case it is often fatal. Some forms are highly contagious.

6. **hernia** _____

The protrusion of a loop or knuckle of an organ or tissue through an abnormal opening. There are several classifications of hernias. The most common types follow.

7. **abdominal hernia** _____

The protrusion of some internal body structure through the abdominal wall.

8. **hiatal hernia** _____

The protrusion of the stomach above the diaphragm. There are both a sliding hiatal hernia and a paraesophageal hiatal hernia.

9. **sliding hiatal hernia** _____

A hernia in which the stomach and a section of esophagus which joins the stomach slide up into the chest through what is called the hiatus (gap/passage).

10. **paraesophageal hiatal hernia** _____

A hernia in which part of the stomach squeezes through the hiatus, but the esophagus and stomach stay in their regular locations. Of concern is that the stomach can become strangled/have its blood supply shut down.

II. **SPELLING.**
Determine if the following words are spelled correctly. If the spelling is correct, leave the word as it has already been entered. If the spelling is incorrect, provide the correct spelling.

1. gastritis _____   2. halitosus _____

3. hepatitus _____   4. gastrenteritis _____

5. gastroesophageal reflex disease _____

III. **MATCHING.**
Match the correct term to the definition.

1. ____ The protrusion of a loop or knuckle of an organ or tissue through an abnormal opening.

2. ____ A hernia in which part of the stomach squeezes through the hiatus but the esophagus and stomach stay in their regular locations.

3. ____ The protrusion of the stomach above the diaphragm.

4. ____ A hernia in which the stomach and a section of esophagus which joins the stomach slide up into the chest through the hiatus.

5. ____ The protrusion of some internal body structure through the abdominal wall.

A. paraesophageal hiatal
B. hiatal
C. hernia
D. abdominal
E. sliding hiatal

Gastrointestinal Disorders – Lesson 5

I. **TERMINOLOGY.**
   Enter each term in the space provided. Read the definition and description for each term.

1. **inguinal hernia** _____

A hernia into the inguinal canal. There are both direct and indirect inguinal hernias.

2. **umbilical hernia** _____

Protrusion of part of the intestine through the umbilicus.

3. **Hirschsprung disease** _____

Congenital megacolon, or a dilatation and hypertrophy of the colon due to the sustained contraction of the muscles of the rectosigmoid.

4. **hypertrophy** _____

The enlargement of an organ due to an increase in the size of its cells.

5. **Ileus** _____

The temporary cessation of intestinal peristalsis, which often leads to obstruction. A common type is adynamic ileus.

6. **adynamic ileus** _____

A suspension of peristalsis because of paralysis or atony (lack of normal muscle tone or strength). This can be the result of drugs, toxemia, trauma, or surgery.

7. **inflammatory bowel disease** _____

This can be used to describe a variety of bowel disorders which are inflammatory in nature, whose etiology cannot be directly determined. There are two common types of inflammatory bowel disease which you should know: Crohn disease & ulcerative colitis.

8. **Crohn disease** _____

It is not known what causes Crohn disease; it can affect any part of the GI tract from the mouth to the anus, but is especially common in the ileocecal area. It frequently leads to obstruction and fistula and abscess formation.

9. **ulcerative colitis** _____

A chronic, nonspecific, inflammatory, and ulcerative disease that arises in the colonic mucosa and usually involves the rectum. Its etiology is also unknown and it is most often manifested by bloody diarrhea.

10. **intussusception** _____

This occurs when a segment of bowel advances and protrudes into the segment distal to it.

II. MULTIPLE CHOICE.
Choose the best answer.

1. Protrusion of the intestine through the bellybutton.
   - ⃝ imbilical hernia
   - ⃝ umbilical hernia
   - ⃝ umbilicus hernia
   - ⃝ imbicilic hernia

2. When a segment of bowel protrudes into the segment distal to it.
   - ⃝ intususception
   - ⃝ intissusception
   - ⃝ intussuception
   - ⃝ intussusception

3. A dilatation and hypertrophy of the colon due to the sustained contraction of the muscles of the rectosigmoid.
   - ⃝ Hirshsprung disease
   - ⃝ Hirschsprung disease
   - ⃝ Huirshsprung disease
   - ⃝ Hurschsprung disease

4. A subacute chronic enteritis of unknown cause.
   - ⃝ Crohn disease
   - ⃝ Crohan disease
   - ⃝ Corhn Disease
   - ⃝ Croahn Disease

5. A suspension of peristalsis because of paralysis or atony.
   - ⃝ a dynamic ilius
   - ⃝ adynamic ilius
   - ⃝ adynamic ileus
   - ⃝ adynamac ileus

III. **TRUE/FALSE.**
   Mark the following true or false.

   1. Intussusception is the enlargement of an organ due to an increase in the size of its cells.
      ○ true
      ○ false

   2. The cause of ulcerative colitis is unknown and it is most often manifested by bloody diarrhea.

      ○ true
      ○ false

   3. There are both direct and indirect inguinal hernias.
      ○ true
      ○ false

   4. Hypertrophy is the shrinking of an organ due to a decrease in the size of its cells.
      ○ true
      ○ false

   5. The permanent cessation of intestinal movement which can lead to obstruction is called ileus.

      ○ true
      ○ false

Gastrointestinal Disorders – Lesson 6

   I. **TERMINOLOGY.**
   Enter each term in the space provided. Read the definition and description for each term.

   1. **irritable bowel syndrome** _____

   Intermittent or constant abdominal distress and bowel dysfunction which has no demonstrable cause.

   2. **jaundice** _____

   A syndrome characterized by the bile pigment in the skin, mucous membranes, and sclerae with a resulting yellow appearance. There are many types of jaundice and most of these indicate a problem with the liver.

   3. **leukoplakia** _____

   A white patch on a mucous membrane that will not rub off. This occurs in the oral mucosa and is considered to be a premalignant (precancerous) lesion common in smokers.

4. **malabsorption** _____

Impaired intestinal absorption of nutrients. If the body is not absorbing nutrients properly, it can quickly result in an insufficiency of necessary nutrients. The combination of weight loss, diarrhea, and anemia indicate malabsorption.

5. **mumps** _____

An acute, highly contagious viral disease which causes painful enlargement of the salivary glands. Primarily infects children under age 15.

6. **obstruction** _____

The state or condition of being clogged or blocked. In gastroenterology it usually refers to a complete arrest or serious impairment to the passage of intestinal contents. You can probably imagine the physical manifestations of obstructions. They are generally caused by adhesions, hernias, tumors, foreign bodies, inflammatory bowel disease, fecal impaction, and volvulus.

7. **pancreatitis** _____

Inflammation of the pancreas.

8. **parasites** _____

A plant or animal which lives upon or within another living organism at whose expense it obtains an advantage. It is not uncommon for a parasite to be present in foods that are consumed, and they are also communicable via person-to-person contact.

9. **Giardia** _____

An intestinal protozoa that has a large sucking disc which adheres to the microvilli of the intestinal walls. There are many different kinds of parasites. However, except for Giardia, they are much more common in Africa and rarely impact Western medicine.

10. **giardiasis** _____

The infection that occurs with the presence of the Giardia parasite.

II. **MULTIPLE CHOICE.**
   Choose the best answer.

   1. Inflammation of the pancreas.
      ◯ pancreasitis
      ◯ pancreatitis
      ◯ pancretitis
      ◯ pancreacitis

   2. A common parasite.
      ◯ Geardia
      ◯ Giardea
      ◯ giardia
      ◯ Giardia

3. Impaired absorption of nutrients.

  ○ dysabsorption
  ○ mallabsorption
  ○ malabsorption
  ○ mallabsorpshun

4. A white patch on a mucous membrane that will not rub off.

  ○ leukoplasia
  ○ leucoplakia
  ○ leucoplacia
  ○ leukoplakia

5. A yellowish appearance.

  ○ jaundice
  ○ jauntice
  ○ jaundace
  ○ Janduace

III. MATCHING.
Match the correct term to the definition.

1. ____ The infection which occurs with the presence of the Giardia parasite.

2. ____ Intermittent or constant abdominal distress and bowel dysfunction which has no demonstrable cause.

3. ____ An acute, highly contagious viral disease which causes painful enlargement of the salivary glands.

4. ____ A plant or animal which lives upon or within another living organism at whose expense it obtains an advantage.

5. ____ The state or condition of being clogged or blocked.

A. mumps
B. giardiasis
C. irritable bowel syndrome
D. obstruction
E. parasite

Gastrointestinal Disorders – Lesson 7

I. **TERMINOLOGY.**
   Enter each term in the space provided. Read the definition and description for each term.

1. **peptic ulcer disease** _____

Inflammation and ulceration in the duodenum and stomach caused by gastric acid juice. Peptic ulcer occurs only if the stomach secretes acid.

2. **Barrett esophagus** _____

Barrett esophagus is a chronic peptic ulcer of the esophagus and is commonly seen in medical reports.

3. **peritonitis** _____

Inflammation of the peritoneum. Symptoms include abdominal pain and tenderness, constipation, vomiting, and moderate fever. Peritonitis sometimes follows abdominal surgery, such as an appendectomy.

4. **pharyngitis** _____

Inflammation of the pharynx. This is the most common etiology of a sore throat.

5. **polyp** _____

This refers to any mass of tissue that arises from the bowel wall and protrudes into the lumen. They may be either sessile or pedunculated. They vary considerably in size and histologic (microscopic tissue structure) characteristics.

6. **sessile** _____

Sessile means attached by a base.

7. **pedunculated** _____

Pedunculated means attached by a stem-like structure or stalk.

8. **prolapse** _____

The falling down or sinking of a part. This pathology can affect the GI system through anal prolapse and rectal prolapse (where skin of the anus and mucosa of the rectum protrude through the anus).

9. **pruritus ani** _____

Pruritus means itching. Pruritus ani is intense, chronic itching in the anal region.

10. **Schatzki ring** _____

A 2–4 mm mucosal structure, probably congenital in nature, which causes a ring-like narrowing of the lower esophagus.

11. **ulcers** _____

A defect or excavation of the surface of an organ or tissue. There are many kinds of ulcers (peptic ulcer disease, stress ulcers, ulcerative colitis, etc.), many causes for ulcers, and many treatments for ulcers.

12. **volvulus** _____

Intestinal obstruction that is due to a knotting or twisting of the bowel.

II. **SPELLING.**
Determine if the following words are spelled correctly. If the spelling is correct, leave the word as it has already been entered. If the spelling is incorrect, provide the correct spelling.

1. pruritis ani _____

2. pharyngitis _____

3. Barrett esophagus _____

4. pepic _____

5. ulcer _____

III. **MULTIPLE CHOICE.**
Choose the best answer.

1. A (◯Schatzki,◯Shatzki) ring is likely congenital in nature.

2. A (◯volvulus,◯prolapse) is an intestinal obstruction.

3. Peritonitis is inflammation of the (◯perineum,◯peritoneum).

4. A (◯pedunculated,◯sessile) polyp is attached by a base.

5. Any mass of tissue that arises from the bowel wall and protrudes into the lumen is referred to as a (◯polyp,◯ulcer).

Bacteria Affecting the Digestive System

You may have noticed that specific common parasites and protozoa are responsible for the etiology of several gastrointestinal problems. Even more common in the causation for the symptoms and diseases of this system are bacteria. The term *bacteria* is actually a plural form of the word *bacterium*, which in human medicine is a pathogenic microorganism whose cell is enclosed in a cell wall. Because these are responsible for a great number of gastrointestinal problems, and because of their unusual spelling rules, they are being discussed slightly separate from the rest of the disease processes. Only those bacteria that affect the digestive system will be discussed here.

The names for individual bacteria are sometimes long and difficult to remember. In addition, they have unique capitalization requirements. The first name or family of bacteria represented is capitalized. The second name is the species, which is not capitalized. Sometimes only the family will be given and the individual species will not.

I. FILL IN THE BLANK.
Enter the word in the blank provided.

1. *Campylobacter* _____

2. *Clostridium botulinum* _____

3. *Clostridium difficile* _____

4. *Clostridium perfringens* _____

5. *Clostridium tetani* _____

6. *Escherichia coli* _____

7. *Enterobacter* _____

8. *Helicobacter pylori* _____

9. *Salmonella* _____

10. *Shigella boydii* _____

11. *Shigella dysenteriae* _____

12. *Staphylococcus aureus* _____

II. SPELLING.
Determine if the following words are spelled correctly. If the spelling is correct, leave the word as it has already been entered. If the spelling is incorrect, provide the correct spelling.

1. Clostrideum perfringens _____

2. Shigella Dysenteriae _____

3. Escherichia coli _____

4. Salmonella _____

5. Clostridium dificile _____

6. Staphylococus aureus _____

7. Camalobacter _____

8. helicobacter pylori _____

9. Shigela boydii _____

10. Anterobacter _____

Unit 6
Respiratory System

Respiratory System – Introduction

The respiratory system works in close combination with the circulatory system to provide a constant supply of oxygen (O_2) to every cell in the body and to remove all gaseous waste (carbon dioxide or CO_2) from the body. Its structures allow life-giving gas exchange between the blood and the atmosphere. This is the primary function of respiration.

The respiratory system is responsible for important secondary functions as well. These include vocalization (speech), or the production of sound as air passes over the vocal cords; assistance with abdominal compression that occurs during micturition (urination), defecation, and parturition (childbirth); and the natural reflexes of coughing and sneezing, which assure that the respiratory system is kept clean.

Highlights

The respiratory system performs the following important functions:

- Gas exchange between blood and atmosphere
- Speech
- Assistance with abdominal compression
- Natural reflexes (sneezing/coughing)

Respiration

The respiratory tract begins at the lips and nostrils and ends at the lungs. The respiratory system also consists of structures that are important in digestion, such as the mouth and the pharynx.

The respiratory system is broken down into the upper respiratory system and the lower respiratory system. The upper respiratory system is "all in your head" (and upper throat) and is comprised of the nasal cavity, nares, larynx, hard palate, soft palate, and pharynx. The lower respiratory system begins with the trachea and encompasses the lungs and bronchi.

The Respiratory System

Respiration is an involuntary process controlled by the brain, and it consists of two basic functions:

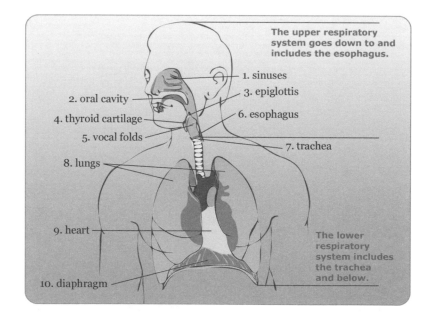

The upper respiratory system goes down to and includes the esophagus.

1. sinuses
2. oral cavity
3. epiglottis
4. thyroid cartilage
5. vocal folds
6. esophagus
7. trachea
8. lungs
9. heart
10. diaphragm

The lower respiratory system includes the trachea and below.

1. **Ventilation**: This is the process of breathing in and out.
   a. Inspiration: Inspiration occurs when the diaphragm (the musculomembranous partition separating the abdominal and thoracic cavities and the major inspiratory muscle) moves to create a slight vacuum in the chest cavity, allowing the lungs to expand and draw air from the airway inward to the lungs.
   b. Expiration: At the end of this cycle expiration occurs. This is when the chest wall relaxes and the lungs contract to expel air. During a very deep inspiration, the capacity of the chest cavity is maximized. All of the muscles—the scalenus anterior, pectoralis major, and sternocleidomastoid—contract to elevate the ribs. You can feel this process yourself by placing your hands on your ribcage and taking a deep breath. Then, with your nose plugged and your mouth tightly shut, attempt to suck in air. You should not be able to feel your ribs elevate as in the previous exercise.

2. **Diffusion**: This is the process of becoming widely spread. Specifically, oxygen is carried to every cell of the body by passing first through the pulmonary alveoli and then to the blood. Finally, carbon dioxide is released from the cells back into the blood, carried through the pulmonary alveoli, and released back out of the tract and into the atmosphere.

I. **FILL IN THE BLANK.**
   Enter the bolded terms in the space provided.

   1. **diaphragm** _____

   2. **epiglottis** _____

   3. **esophagus** _____

   4. **heart** _____

   5. **lungs** _____

   6. **oral cavity** _____

   7. **sinuses** _____

   8. **thyroid cartilage** _____

   9. **trachea** _____

   10. **vocal folds** _____

II. FILL IN THE BLANK.

Refer to the image and enter the terms corresponding to the following numbers. Use the words in the box to fill in the blanks.

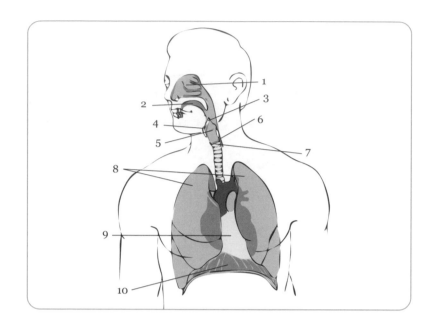

1. _____

2. _____

3. _____

4. _____

5. _____

6. _____

7. _____

8. _____

9. _____

10. _____

thyroid cartilage
heart
epiglottis
trachea
diaphragm
sinuses
esophagus
vocal folds
oral cavity
lungs

Gross Respiratory Anatomy

Several physical requirements must be met in order for ventilation and diffusion to be effective. First, the actual structures in which the gaseous exchange takes place must have thin, permeable walls (or membranes) so that diffusion can easily occur. In addition, these membranes must be kept moist so that the oxygen and carbon dioxide can be dissolved in water. A rich blood supply is also a necessary factor. Furthermore, the gaseous exchange must take place deeply enough within the body so that the incoming air can be made sufficiently warm. Lastly, a pump must be present in order to constantly replenish the air.

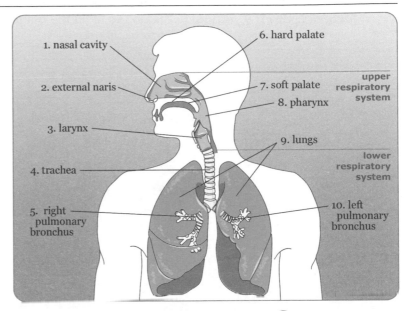

Some structures are part of both the respiratory and digestive systems. For the most part, the basic structures of the respiratory system should not be difficult for you to learn, but a couple of items should be noted. First, the external *naris* refers to one nostril. The plural form is *nares* and it is more commonly used. *Bronchus* is also singular, with the plural form being *bronchi*. Here, too, the plural is the more commonly used form.

Here is a slightly different diagram of the respiratory system. Note the nasal cavity (which houses some of the sinuses), the external naris, the hard and soft palates (within the oral cavity), and the right and left pulmonary bronchi.

Some structures are part of more than one system. For example, the oral cavity (mouth) is the beginning point of the digestive system AND an important point for air entry into the respiratory system.

I. FILL IN THE BLANK.

In the blanks below, refer to the image and enter the term corresponding to the following numbers. Use the word(s) in the box to fill in the blanks.

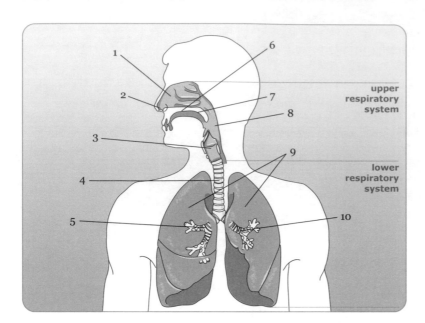

1. _____

2. _____

3. _____

4. _____

5. _____

6. _____

7. _____

8. _____

9. _____

10. _____

external naris
left pulmonary bronchus
pharynx
nasal cavity
hard palate
trachea
right pulmonary bronchus
lungs
larynx
soft palate

Determine if the anatomical part belongs to the upper or lower respiratory system. Fill in the blank with either "upper" or "lower."

1. lungs _____

2. soft palate _____

3. pharynx _____

4. right pulmonary bronchus _____

5. nasal cavity _____

6. larynx _____

7. left pulmonary bronchus _____

8. trachea _____

9. hard palate _____

10. external naris _____

Nasal Cavity

Air can be taken in simultaneously through the oral and nasal cavities. It can also be taken in through only the oral cavity or only the nasal cavity just as effectively. Unless there is some obstruction, people take in most of their oxygen through the nasal cavity. This is divided into two equal cavities by the nasal septum that serves as the partition. The perpendicular ethmoid and vomer bones, along with septal cartilage, make up the nasal septum. Each side opens into the external nares (nostrils). There are also internal (posterior) nares or choanae (singular choana) that link the external nares to the nasopharynx.

Highlights

Functions of the nasal cavity:

1. Warm, moisten, and clean air
2. Sense of smell
3. Sound resonation (singing/speech)

The bones that make up the nose are the frontal, nasal, palatine, maxillae, and conchae (also called turbinates). The conchae, or turbinate, bones create a passageway for air; this passage is called the meatus. Air enters through the external naris, travels up the meatus (which is often designated in sections—anterior, middle, posterior), passes through the choana, and into the nasopharynx.

The nasal cavity itself serves three major functions:

1. It warms, moistens, and cleans the inhaled air. Epithelium refers to the covering of various surfaces of the body, both internal and external, including the linings of small cavities and vessels. The nasal epithelia cover the conchae (turbinate bones) and serve to warm, moisten, and clean the air that is taken in. The epithelial lining contains many blood vessels that enable it to warm the air. These vessels are the source of nosebleeds (medical term—epistaxis). Nasal hairs are also present in this lining and sometimes extend outside the nostrils. These are actually filters for microscopic particles that might otherwise be inhaled.

2. It is the olfactory center. One of the senses is also an integral function of the nasal cavity—the sense of smell. The medical term for this is *olfaction*. The olfactory epithelia are located in the upper posterior part of the nasal cavity and are associated with the reception of odors. The olfactory system protects the body by alerting it to harmful contaminants in the air, as well as to potential dangers in foods. Of course, it is responsible for certain pleasant associations: the smell of baking cookies or sizzling hamburgers, the perfume of flowers, or the scent of aftershave.

3. The third function of the nasal cavity is related to sound production. The nasal cavity serves as a resonating chamber for the voice. As such, it prolongs and intensifies the sound vibrations created by the voice box (larynx), thus aiding in speech production and enhancing vocal music.

I. **TERMINOLOGY.**
   Enter each term in the space provided. Read the definition and description for each term.

   1. **nasal septum** _____
   The partition that divides the two equal cavities of the nose.

   2. **perpendicular ethmoid** _____
   One bone that makes up the nasal septum.

   3. **vomer** _____
   One bone that makes up the nasal septum.

   4. **external nares** _____
   The nostrils.

   5. **choanae** _____
   Internal nares that link the external nares to the nasopharynx.

   6. **conchae bones** _____
   Also called turbinate bones, they create a passageway for the air.

   7. **meatus** _____
   The passage created by the conchae where air flows.

   8. **nasopharynx** _____
   The nasal portion of the pharynx.

II. TRUE/FALSE.
Mark the following true or false.

1. The medical term for the sense of smell is olfaction.

   ○ true
   ○ false

2. The nasal cavity has nothing to do with sound production in the human body.

   ○ true
   ○ false

3. Epithelia cover the conchae to warm, moisten, and clean air taken in through the nose.

   ○ true
   ○ false

Sinus Cavities

Certain bones of the face are configured to create air spaces. These interosseous spaces are called the paranasal sinuses. They are named after the bones that create them—maxillary, frontal, sphenoid, and ethmoidal (or ethmoid). They communicate with the nasal cavity and assist in respiration by warming and moistening inspired air. They also allow for lessening the weight of the skull without compromising its strength. Unfortunately, these warm, moist sinuses are susceptible to infection. Sinus infections are quite common, so familiarize yourself with the location and names of the various sinus cavities.

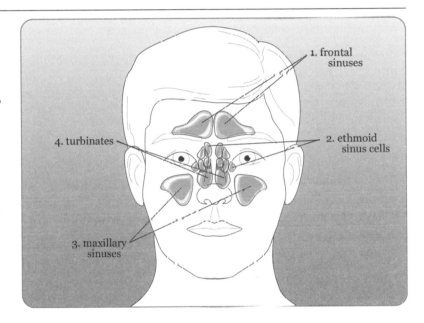

1. frontal sinuses

2. ethmoid sinus cells

3. maxillary sinuses

4. turbinates

FILL IN THE BLANK.
Use the word(s) in the box to fill in the blanks.

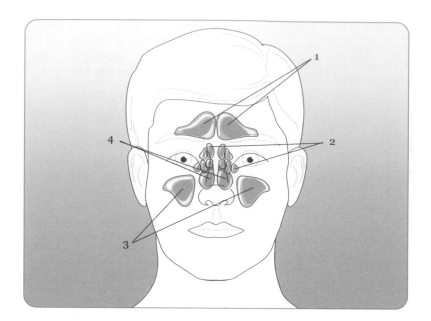

1. _____

2. _____

3. _____

4. _____

maxillary sinuses
turbinates
ethmoid sinus cells
frontal sinuses

Pharynx

The pharynx is the passageway that connects the nasal and oral cavities to the larynx. It is divided into three distinct regions based upon function:

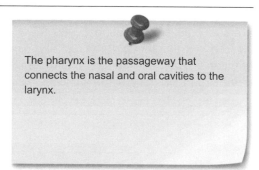

The pharynx is the passageway that connects the nasal and oral cavities to the larynx.

1. First is the **nasopharynx**. This is only respiratory in function. It is the uppermost portion of the pharynx. The paired auditory, or eustachian, tubes connect the nasopharynx to the cavities of the middle ear. The pharyngeal tonsils, more commonly called adenoids, are found in the posterior wall of this cavity.

2. Second is the **oropharynx**. This is the middle portion of the pharynx. Palatine tonsils are located at the back and side (posterolateral) wall of the oropharynx, and lingual tonsils are found at the base of the tongue. Tonsils are small, rounded masses of tissue. When used generically, (as in "he had his tonsils out") the reference is to the palatine tonsils. Tonsillitis, an infection of the palatine or lingual tonsils, can occur even after a tonsillectomy (excision or removal of the tonsils).

3. The third and final portion of the pharynx is the **laryngopharynx**. This is the lowermost portion. The respiratory and digestive tracts diverge here at the laryngopharynx. Food and fluids enter the esophagus, and air goes into the larynx.

I. FILL IN THE BLANK.
Using the word/word parts in the box, fill in the blanks.

1. The respiratory and digestive tracts diverge at the

   _____.

2. The _____ is only respiratory in function.

3. The passageway that connects the nasal and oral cavities to the

   larynx is the _____.

4. The _____ is where the palatine tonsils are found.

pharynx
oropharynx
laryngopharynx
nasopharynx

Larynx and Trachea

The larynx is the entrance to the lower respiratory tract. Its three main functions are:

1. Control of the airflow between the pharynx and the trachea.
2. Prevent food or fluid from getting into the trachea and thus into the lungs upon swallowing.
3. Produce the sound vibrations. This last function gives rise to the term *voice box*. Another term for the voice box is the *glottis*.

The larynx is composed of nine cartilages, the largest being called the thyroid cartilage. This is more prominent in males than in females and is also called the *Adam's apple*.

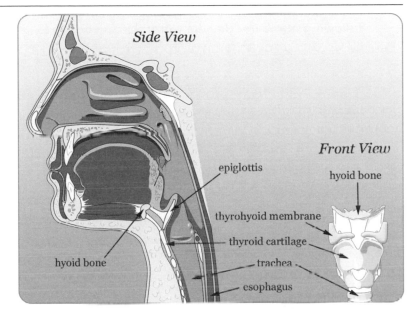

The lower end of the larynx is made up of ring-shaped cricoid cartilage. A pair of arytenoid cartilages are situated above the cricoid and are attached to the vocal cords. The vocal cords are actually two pairs of strong connective tissue bands stretched across the upper opening of the larynx. They are called the true vocal cords and the false vocal cords. The false vocal cords (also called ventricular folds) support the true vocal cords but are not actually used in sound production. The true vocal cords vibrate to cause sound as air moves across them.

The larynx opens at its lower end into the trachea (also called the windpipe), a rigid tube that is approximately 4.5 inches in length, which connects the larynx to the bronchi. A series of 16 to 20 C-shaped hyaline cartilage rings make up the wall of the trachea. The open part of the C is at the back of the trachea and is covered by connective tissue and smooth muscle. This allows for the trachea to be rigid but flexible, yet still allows for the lumen of the tube to be permanently open.

Two additional terms need to be introduced at this point. The epiglottis is the flap of cartilage that covers the windpipe (trachea) when swallowing occurs, preventing food and liquids from entering the trachea. The small conical piece of flesh that hangs down from the posterior portion of the soft palate is called the uvula. It is a remnant left as the soft palate forms during fetal development. It is used in the production of sounds in some languages other than English.

When you inhale tiny dust particles, they stick to the mucous layer of the trachea, and the cilia (minute, hair-like processes) sweep those particles upwards to the pharynx where they are removed by coughing. As you will discover below, smoking and air pollution destroy the cilia, thus allowing contaminants to enter the lungs.

I. **FILL IN THE BLANK.**
   Enter the bolded terms in the space provided.

1. **epiglottis** _____

2. **esophagus** _____

3. **hyoid bone** _____

4. **thyrohyoid membrane** _____

5. **thyroid cartilage** _____

6. **trachea** _____

II. **FILL IN THE BLANK.**
   In the blanks provided below, refer to the image and enter the term corresponding to the following numbers. Use the word(s) in the box to fill in the blanks.

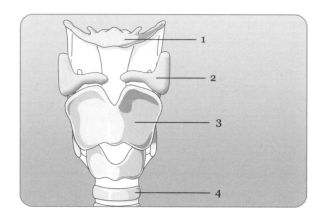

1. _____

2. _____

3. _____

4. _____

| thyroid cartilage |
| trachea |
| thyrohyoid membrane |
| hyoid bone |

III. FILL IN THE BLANK.

In the blanks provided below, refer to the image and enter the term corresponding to the following numbers. Use the word(s) in the box to fill in the blanks.

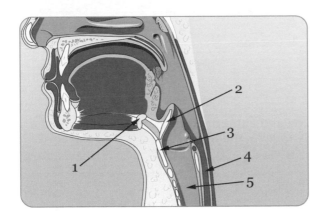

1. _____

2. _____

3. _____

4. _____

5. _____

esophagus
hyoid bone
trachea
thyroid cartilage
epiglottis

Bronchi

The trachea bifurcates, or divides, into two branches at its most distal portion and forms the bronchi. The bifurcation is reinforced by a cartilaginous plate called the carina.

At the bifurcation of the trachea, the respiratory tract divides into a right and left pulmonary bronchus. These structures are called bronchial trees because they are composed of respiratory tubes that branch off and get progressively smaller in diameter. Like the trachea, each bronchus is made up of cartilaginous rings to keep the lumen open as it goes into the lung. As the branches get smaller, they are called secondary bronchi and segmental (or tertiary) bronchi. (The term *tertiary* actually means third in order.) The bronchi then branch into even smaller tubules called bronchioles.

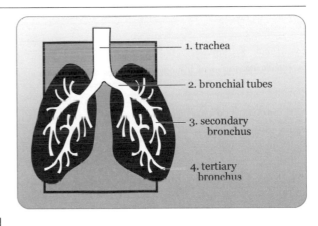

1. trachea

2. bronchial tubes

3. secondary bronchus

4. tertiary bronchus

Many terminal bronchioles deep in the lungs mark the end of the respiratory tract proper. The terminal bronchioles do continue to branch into alveolar ducts that lead into alveolar sacs containing individual alveoli, the basic functional units of the respiratory system. Through them the exchange between alveolar gas and pulmonary capillary blood takes place. Each lung contains an estimated 350 million alveoli.

I. FILL IN THE BLANK.
Enter the bolded terms in the space provided.

1. **bronchial tubes** _____

2. **secondary bronchus** _____

3. **tertiary bronchus** _____

4. **trachea** _____

II. FILL IN THE BLANK.
In the blanks provided below, refer to the image and enter the term corresponding to the following numbers. Use the word(s) in the box to fill in the blanks.

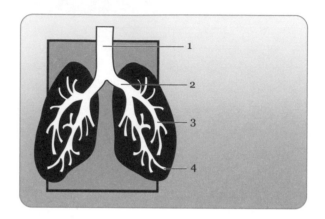

1. _____

2. _____

3. _____

4. _____

secondary bronchus
trachea
tertiary bronchus
bronchial tubes

Lungs

The lungs themselves are large soft organs within the thoracic cavity. The lungs are separated from each other by the mediastinal space and its contents, which constitutes the mediastinum. It contains several organs and structures, including the heart, trachea, esophagus, lymph nodes, nerves, major circulatory branches, and more. Among the major circulatory branches are the aorta and the superior vena cava. You will be exposed to these further in the lessons on the cardiovascular system. The left lung is slightly smaller than the right and is designated as having a superior (upper) and inferior (lower) lobe.

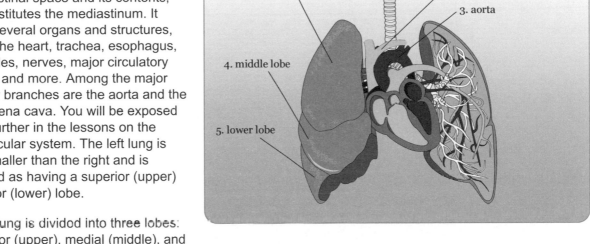

The right lung is divided into three lobes: the superior (upper), medial (middle), and inferior (lower). The lobes of both lungs are then further divided into smaller lobules that contain the alveoli.

The lungs are surrounded by the pleura, which is a serous membrane that lines the thoracic cavity and encloses the entire space of the pleural cavity. It is divided into two sections, the right and the left, to coincide with the right and left lungs.

The pleura is further divided into two parts: the visceral pleura adheres to the outer surface of the lung, and the parietal pleura lines the thoracic wall and thoracic side of the diaphragm.

I. FILL IN THE BLANK.

In the blanks provided below, refer to the image and enter the term corresponding to the following numbers. Use the word(s) in the box to fill in the blanks.

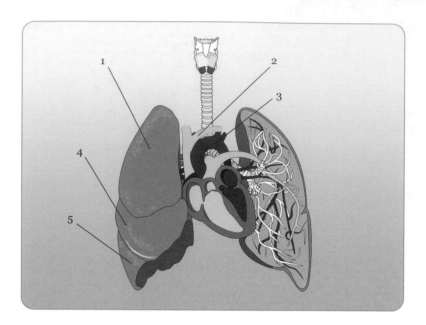

1. _____

2. _____

3. _____

4. _____

5. _____

superior vena cava
middle lobe
aorta
upper lobe
lower lobe

Respiratory Terminology

Term	Definition
septum	Partition between the two sides of the nasal cavity.
ethmoid	Perforated like a sieve, such as the ethmoid bone.
vomer	Bone of the nasal septum.
choana(e)	Link from external nares to nasopharynx.
turbinates	Another name for conchae.
meatus	Passageway in the body, especially an opening on the surface.
epithelium	Lining of small cavities.
epistaxis	Nosebleed.
olfaction	Sense of smell.
olfactory epithelia	Lines the olfactory region of the nasal cavity.

paranasal sinuses	Air spaces contained by certain bones of the face.
maxillary sinus	One of the paired paranasal sinuses located in the body of the maxilla.
frontal sinus	One of the paired irregular shaped paranasal sinuses located in the frontal bone.
sphenoid sinus	One of the paired paranasal sinuses in the anterior part of the body of the sphenoid bone.
ethmoidal sinus	One of the paranasal sinuses located within the ethmoid bone.
auditory	Pertaining to the sense of hearing.
eustachian	Tube connecting the nasopharynx to the middle ear.
adenoids	Pharyngeal tonsils.
laryngopharynx	Where the respiratory and digestive systems diverge.
thyroid	Gland situated in the lower part of the front of the neck.
cricoid	Ring-shaped cartilage making up the lower larynx.
arytenoid	Vocal cord cartilage.
bifurcates	Divided into two branches.
bifurcation	Site where a single structure divides into two.
carina	Cartilaginous plate of the trachea.
bronchial tree	Another name for pulmonary bronchus.
tertiary	Third in order.
bronchioles	One of the subdivisions of the branched bronchial tree.
alveolar ducts	Small passages connecting the respiratory bronchioles and the alveolar sacs.
alveoli	Functional units of the respiratory system.
mediastinal space	Space separating the lungs.
mediastinum	Mass of tissues and organs separating the two pleural sacs.
lobules	Division of lung lobes.
pleura	Serous membrane of the thoracic cavity.
visceral	Pleura which is adherent to the outer surface of the lung.
parietal	Pleura that lines the thoracic wall and diaphragm.

Pulmonology

The specialty that deals primarily with chronic, acute, or severe problems of the respiratory system is pulmonology. Upper respiratory system and less acute or severe respiratory complaints are often handled by specialties like ENT and otolaryngology, as well as family practice physicians.

In a hospital setting, the internal medicine department is likely to diagnose, treat, and follow up with patients admitted for respiratory pathology—pneumonia, for example. It is also the case that the respiratory therapy department works with those patients, gauging progress via incentive spirometry (the measurement of the breathing capacity of the lungs), performing such therapeutic measures as percussion and postural drainage, nebulizer treatments, and mist tents. They also work with the physician to evaluate arterial or venous blood gases, primarily oxygen and carbon dioxide. These laboratory studies will be addressed in the relevant unit of the program.

As you might expect, there is considerable crossover between pulmonology and other medical specialties. Because of the close interaction between the heart and the lungs, cardiology reports of one kind or another will make reference to respiratory words and phrases. Many infectious diseases involve the lungs so that particular specialty is also one that uses pulmonary terminology. Chest x-rays are a routine preoperative practice for any major surgery. Thus, terms associated with the respiratory system appear in a variety of different specialties.

It is also the case that the respiratory system is consistently affected by viruses, such as those which produce the common cold and flu, and by allergies. Especially in a clinic or doctor's office situation, problems associated with the respiratory structures, components, and disease processes are very commonly evaluated and treated.

Before continuing on, please review the terms found in this introductory section.

I. **TERMINOLOGY.**
   Enter each term in the space provided. Read the definition and description for each term.

   1. **ventilation** _____
   Process of the exchange of air between the lungs and the ambient air.

   2. **inspiration** _____
   Drawing air inward to the lungs.

   3. **diaphragm** _____
   Partition that separates the abdominal and thoracic cavities.

   4. **expiration** _____
   The relaxation of the chest wall.

   5. **diffusion** _____
   Process of becoming widely spread.

   6. **pulmonary alveoli** _____
   Small outpouchings along the walls of the alveolar sacs where gas exchange takes place.

   7. **pulmonology** _____
   Specialty that deals primarily with problems of the respiratory system.

   8. **incentive spirometry** _____
   Measurement of the breathing capacity of the lungs.

II. MULTIPLE CHOICE.
Choose the best answer.

1. Science concerned with the anatomy, physiology, and pathology of the lungs.
   - ○ breathology
   - ○ pulmonology
   - ○ respirology
   - ○ biology

2. Drawing air inward to the lungs.
   - ○ expiration
   - ○ ventilation
   - ○ incentive spirometry
   - ○ inspiration

3. The process of becoming widely spread, as in oxygen to every cell.
   - ○ diffusion
   - ○ inspiration
   - ○ defecation
   - ○ expiration

4. The process of the exchange of air between the lungs and the ambient air.
   - ○ separation
   - ○ diffusion
   - ○ aspiration
   - ○ ventilation

5. Measurement of the breathing capacity of the lungs.
   - ○ incentive spirometry
   - ○ incentive ventilation
   - ○ micturition
   - ○ incentive diffusion

6. The musculomembranous partition that separates the abdominal and thoracic cavities.

○ omentum
○ partition
○ diaphragm
○ parietal

7. When the chest wall relaxes.

○ expiration
○ expires
○ inspires
○ ventilation

Respiratory Symptoms

The respiratory system, as mentioned, is susceptible to disease. Its proper function is also essential to the sustaining of life. Much like the digestive system, respiration can be greatly impacted by what we choose to take into our lungs. This can be either deliberate, such as cigarette smoking, or incidental, such as air pollution. A serious problem with respiration usually requires hospitalization. Thus, in an acute care setting, many patients are admitted for treatment of respiratory pathology.

As with any disease process, there will be a symptom or series of symptoms that enable a healthcare professional to determine the etiology. The list on the following page comprises only the most common symptoms. Commit the following terms to memory.

I. **TERMINOLOGY.**
   Enter each term in the space provided. Read the definition and description for each term.

   1. **chest pain** _____

   Any discomfort in the thoracic cavity.

   2. **clubbing** _____

   Enlargement of the ends of the fingers and toes with loss of the nailbed angle. This can be an indication of several pulmonary disorders and is usually examined in conjunction with cyanosis and edema.

   3. **congestion** _____

   Excessive or abnormal accumulation of fluid (such as mucus in the sinuses).

   4. **cough** _____

   A sudden, noisy expulsion of air from the lungs. This is a reflex to keep the airway free of foreign matter.

   5. **cyanosis** _____

   Bluish discoloration, particularly of the nailbeds and perioral area. Again, this may be seen in conjunction with clubbing and edema.

6. **dyspnea** _____

Difficulty breathing.

7. **hemoptysis** _____

Coughing up blood or bloodstained sputum, usually due to bleeding somewhere in the respiratory tract.

8. **hiccup (hiccough)** _____

An involuntary spasmodic contraction of the diaphragm that occurs on inspiration and results in a distinctive sound. You may sometimes see this spelled "hiccough."

9. **malaise** _____

A vague feeling of bodily discomfort and fatigue, not necessarily related specifically to respiratory function.

10. **sputum** _____

Matter that is ejected from the lungs, bronchi, and trachea through the mouth. The consistency of this matter can be a major factor in determining the pathology of a respiratory problem. Sputum can be watery and clear, purulent (containing pus), viscous (thick), or contain blood, to name a few variations. Its color may also be significant–clear, white, yellow, green, brown, or combinations thereof.

11. **purulent** _____

Containing pus.

12. **rales** _____

Usually pronounced "rawls" (but sometimes "rails" or "rals"—rhyming with "pals"). These are discontinuous nonmusical sounds heard primarily during inspiration. They are also called crackles.

13. **rhonchi** _____

Continuous dry rattling sounds in the throat or bronchial tube due to a partial obstruction.

14. **stridor** _____

A musical sound, heard with a stethoscope on inspiration

15. **tachypnea** _____

Shortness of breath. Excessive rapidity of respiration or quick, shallow breathing.

16. **wheezing** _____

Whistling or wheezing noises associated with breathing; a telltale symptom of asthma.

II. FILL IN THE BLANK.
Determine if the word is a body part or symptom. Fill in the blanks with 'part' or 'symptom.'

1. tachypnea _____

2. larynx _____

3. hemoptysis _____

4. wheezing _____

5. alveoli _____

6. rales _____

7. malaise _____

8. trachea _____

9. uvula _____

10. dyspnea _____

11. bronchus _____

12. clubbing _____

13. lungs _____

14. naris _____

Assessing Respiratory Symptoms

Physicians can determine the cause of a symptom or set of symptoms by several diagnostic methods. Usually the first step to discovery is to obtain the subjective history from the patient, and the second is to conduct a physical examination. To determine a pulmonary disorder on physical examination, a physician will usually use percussion and auscultation.

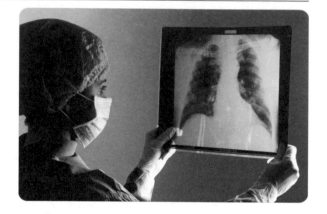

Percussion is the act of striking a part with short, sharp blows. They do this to the front and back of the torso at the level of the thoracic cavity while listening with a stethoscope.

Auscultation is the act of listening for sounds within the body, especially the heart and lungs. Auscultation can reveal to the trained ear the presence of rales, rhonchi, wheezing, stridor, or other sounds. Again, the instrument used for auscultation is the stethoscope.

A serious problem occurs when there is not enough oxygen present in the blood or when the oxygen in the blood is not able to reach a particular part of the body. The deficiency of oxygen in the blood is called hypoxemia or hypoxia. These terms are used interchangeably. The term *anoxia*, although it technically means a total lack of oxygen in the blood, is sometimes used synonymously with hypoxemia.

It is also a dangerous sign when there is an abundance of carbon dioxide present in the blood. This state is called hypercapnia. Pulmonary function tests and arterial blood gas evaluations are utilized to determine if this abnormality is present, and therefore these tests are performed regularly on patients with severe respiratory symptoms. The results of arterial blood gases are represented in a unique way that will be discussed later in the laboratory section of the course.

Radiology examinations, especially chest x-rays, are important in determining the etiology of respiratory failure. In addition, other more invasive tests, such as bronchoscopy (examination of the bronchi with a scope), thoracentesis (the surgical puncture of the chest wall in order to aspirate fluid), biopsies, or major surgery can be utilized if required.

I. FILL IN THE BLANK.
Use the word(s) in the box to fill in the blanks.

thoracentesis
percussion
hypoxemia
bronchoscopy
auscultation
hypoxia
hypercapnia
anoxia

1. Listening for sounds within the body. _____

2. Striking a part with short, sharp blows. _____

3. Deficiency of oxygen in the blood. _____

4. A total lack of oxygen in the blood. _____

5. An abundance of carbon dioxide in the blood.

   _____

6. The surgical puncture of the chest wall in order to aspirate fluid.

   _____

7. Examination of the bronchi with a scope. _____

II. MULTIPLE CHOICE.
Choose the best answer.

1. The noisy expulsion of air from the lungs.
   - ○ congested
   - ○ cough
   - ○ infection
   - ○ auscultation

2. Listening to a body part.
   - ○ percussion
   - ○ thoracentesis
   - ○ palpation
   - ○ auscultation

3. Coughing up blood.
   - ○ anoxia
   - ○ bronchoscopy
   - ○ hemoptysis
   - ○ purulent

4. A deficiency of oxygen in the blood.
   - ○ malaise
   - ○ hypoxemia
   - ○ congestion
   - ○ hyperactive

5. Shortness of breath. Excessive rapidity of respiration or quick, shallow breathing.

○ tachypnea

○ purulent

○ congestion

○ auscultation

6. Too much carbon dioxide present in the blood.

○ hypercapnia

○ tachypnea

○ dyspnea

○ cyanosis

7. A musical sound heard with a stethoscope on inspiration.

○ percussion

○ cyanosis

○ cough

○ stridor

8. Striking a part with short, sharp blows.

○ clubbing

○ auscultation

○ palpation

○ percussion

9. Containing pus.

○ congested

○ cyanotic

○ purulent

○ dyspneic

10. Excessive or abnormal accumulation of fluid.

○ hypoxia

○ hemoptysis

○ cough

○ congestion

11. Bluish discoloration.

○ dyspnea

○ cyanosis

○ bluing

○ hypercapnia

12. Difficulty breathing.

   ○ dyspnea
   ○ cyanosis
   ○ cough
   ○ congested

13. Examination of the bronchi with a scope.

   ○ thoracentesis
   ○ auscultation
   ○ bronchoscopy
   ○ percussion

14. Surgical puncture of the chest wall to aspirate fluid.

   ○ percussion
   ○ thoracentesis
   ○ palpation
   ○ bronchoscopy

Common Respiratory Problems – Lesson 1

The following lists contain many of the more common respiratory problems. While this list is not exhaustive, it is really extensive and will include terms you have already been exposed to in this training program and terms you will be exposed to over and over again throughout the rest of this training program. Read the complete definitions of each term to help differentiate spelling and terms.

I. **TERMINOLOGY.**
   Enter each term In the space provided. Read the definition and description for each term.

   1. **abscess** _____

   A localized collection of pus buried in tissues, organs, or confined spaces.

   2. **adult respiratory distress syndrome (ARDS)** _____

   Chronic respiratory failure associated with various acute pulmonary injuries. It is characterized by pulmonary edema, respiratory distress, and hypoxemia. It is sometimes a complication of major surgery and is accompanied by infection.

   3. **apnea** _____

   Cessation of breathing.

   4. **asphyxia** _____

   Suffocation. This can be deliberate and traumatic, occur as a result of some obstruction of the airway, or due to some other cause.

5. **asthma** _____

This is a condition that is marked by recurrent attacks of paroxysmal dyspnea and it is manifested by wheezing. It can be due to an allergic reaction, strenuous exercise, irritant particles in the air, psychological stresses, or other factors.

6. **paroxysmal** _____

A paroxysm is a sudden recurrence or intensification of symptoms.

7. **atelectasis** _____

Incomplete expansion of a lung, a shrunken or airless lung. This can be either acute or chronic and can be complete or partial. This is determined via a chest x-ray.

8. **bronchiectasis** _____

An irreversible chronic dilation of the bronchi that is usually accompanied by infection. It is manifested by fetid breath and paroxysmal coughing with the expectoration of mucopurulent matter.

9. **fetid** _____

Having a rank or disagreeable smell.

10. **expectoration** _____

The act of coughing up and spitting out materials from the lungs, bronchi, and trachea.

II. **SPELLING.**
   Determine if the following words are spelled correctly. If the spelling is correct, leave the word as it has already been entered. If the spelling is incorrect, provide the correct spelling.

   1. aphyxia _____   2. apnea _____

   3. bronchyectasis _____   4. expecteration _____

   5. paroxysmel _____

III. MULTIPLE CHOICE.
Choose the best answer.

1. A collection of pus in an organ, tissue, or confined space.
   - ⊙ abscess
   - ⊙ absess
   - ⊙ abcess
   - ⊙ absces

2. Chronic respiratory failure associated with various acute pulmonary injuries.
   - ⊙ adult respiritory distress syndrome
   - ⊙ adult respiratory dystress syndrome
   - ⊙ adult respiretory distress syndrome
   - ⊙ adult respiratory distress syndrome

3. A shrunken or airless lung.
   - ⊙ atelectasis
   - ⊙ attelectasis
   - ⊙ atelectiasis
   - ⊙ atellectasis

4. A condition marked by paroxysmal dyspnea and wheezing.
   - ⊙ astma
   - ⊙ asthsma
   - ⊙ azma
   - ⊙ asthma

5. Having a rank or disagreeable smell.
   - ⊙ fetad
   - ⊙ fetid
   - ⊙ phetid
   - ⊙ fecid

Common Respiratory Problems – Lesson 2

I. **TERMINOLOGY.**
   Enter each term in the space provided. Read the definition and description for each term.

   1. **bronchitis** _____

   Inflammation of the mucous membrane lining of the bronchial tubes. Significant contributing factors to this condition are cigarette smoking, pollution, and allergies.

   2. **bronchopneumonia** _____

   An inflammation of the lungs which usually begins in the terminal bronchioles.

   3. **bronchiolitis** _____

   Another name for bronchopneumonia.

   4. **bronchoalveolitis** _____

   Another name for bronchopneumonia.

   5. **bronchopneumonitis** _____

   Another name for bronchopneumonia.

   6. **chronic obstructive pulmonary disease (COPD)** _____

   A generalized term related to persistent airways obstructions. COPD is associated with various combinations of chronic bronchitis, respiratory bronchiolitis, asthma, and/or emphysema. The term "airways obstruction" refers to an increased resistance to airflow during forced expiration.

   7. **coccidioidomycosis** _____

   A fungal disease that infects the respiratory system as a result of the inhalation of spores. Manifested primarily by cold symptoms. Also called "valley fever."

   8. **emphysema** _____

   A pathological accumulation of air in tissues or organs, especially the lungs. In pulmonary emphysema, there is dilatation of the alveoli and destruction of their walls. It is a common cause of disability and eventual death for cigarette smokers.

   9. **empyema** _____

   Accumulation of pus in a cavity of the body. Although there are different types, when the term is used without a qualifier, it refers to thoracic empyema, which is in the pleural space.

   10. **epiglottitis** _____

   Inflammation of the epiglottis.

II. SPELLING.
Determine if the following words are spelled correctly. If the spelling is correct, leave the word as it has already been entered. If the spelling is incorrect, provide the correct spelling.

1. epiglotitis _____   2. bronchiolitis _____

3. bronchipneumonitis _____   4. coccidiodomycosis _____

5. bronchitus _____

III. MATCHING.
Match the correct term to the definition.

1. ____ Another term for bronchopneumonia.

2. ____ Accumulation of pus in a cavity in the body.

3. ____ Generalized term related to persistent airway obstructions.

4. ____ The name given to an inflammation of the lungs which usually begins in the terminal bronchioles.

5. ____ A pathological accumulation of air in tissues or organs, especially the lungs.

A. empyema
B. bronchopneumonia
C. bronchoalveolitis
D. emphysema
E. chronic obstructive airway disease

Common Respiratory Problems – Lesson 3

I. TERMINOLOGY.
Enter each term in the space provided. Read the definition and description for each term.

1. **epistaxis** _____

Nosebleed (hemorrhage from the nose).

2. **hemothorax** _____

A collection of blood in the pleural cavity. This often results from a blunt or penetrating trauma to the chest wall

3. **hyaline membrane disease** _____

This is a disorder usually affecting premature newborns in which the alveoli are lined by a hyaline material. It usually results in extensive atelectasis and is often fatal.

4. **hyperventilation** _____

A state in which there is an increase in the amount of air entering the pulmonary alveoli, which results in a decrease in carbon dioxide tension.

5. **infiltrate** _____

Material deposited in organs or cells which are not normal to it, or in excessive quantities. It is also a sign of acute inflammation.

6. **interstitial lung disease** _____

Interstitial is a term that means pertaining to or situated between parts or in the interspaces of a tissue. There are several types of interstitial lung disease in which there is an abnormal accumulation of many different cell types in the alveoli and bronchioles, which ultimately leads to progressive destruction of the lung.

7. **laryngitis** _____

Inflammation of the larynx. Usually associated with dryness and soreness of the throat, hoarseness, cough, and dysphagia.

8. **papilloma** _____

A papilloma is a benign tumor. In the respiratory system, these are common in children, starting at age one, and can grow exuberantly in the larynx. They are viral in origin and cause hoarseness. They can be removed surgically but tend to recur.

9. **pertussis** _____

An acute, highly contagious infection of the respiratory tract, most frequently seen in young children and characterized by paroxysmal coughing. Also called "whooping cough."

10. **pleural effusion** _____

Excess fluid in the pleural space. The presence of fluid in the pleural space is usually determined by x-ray and almost always requires a thoracentesis.

II. **MULTIPLE CHOICE.**
   Choose the best answer.

1. A collection of blood in the pleural cavity.
   ○ hemathorax
   ○ hemothorax
   ○ hemithorax
   ○ hemiothorax

2. Disease affecting premature newborns.
   ○ hyalin membrane disease
   ○ hyaline membrane disease
   ○ hyeline membrane disease
   ○ hialyne membrane disease

3. Materials deposited in organs or cells which are not normal to it.
   - ◯ infiltrate
   - ◯ infilltrate
   - ◯ inffiltrate
   - ◯ infaltrate

4. A benign tumor.
   - ◯ papiloma
   - ◯ papelloma
   - ◯ papilloma
   - ◯ papillioma

5. Nosebleed.
   - ◯ eppistaxis
   - ◯ epistasis
   - ◯ epistaxis
   - ◯ epostaxis

III. **MULTIPLE CHOICE.**
Choose the best answer.

1. The patient was experiencing (◯hyperventalation, ◯hyperventilation) ; she had an increase in the amount of air entering the pulmonary alveoli.

2. The patient comes in with a past history of (◯interstittial, ◯interstitial) lung disease.

3. Inflammation of the larynx is called (◯larynxitis, ◯laryngitis) .

4. Whooping cough is another name for (◯pertussis, ◯pertusis) .

5. The patient was diagnosed with a (◯plural, ◯pleural) effusion.

Common Respiratory Problems – Lesson 4

I. **TERMINOLOGY.**
Enter each term in the space provided. Read the definition and description for each term.

1. **serous** _____
Fluid that is clear and yellow.

2. **sanguineous** _____
Bloody or blood-tinged fluid.

3. **serosanguineous** _____

Fluid containing both serum and blood.

4. **pleurisy** _____

Inflammation of the pleura. It is usually characterized by pain that is worse with breathing and coughing. The onset is usually sudden.

5. **pneumoconiosis** _____

A condition characterized by the permanent deposition of substantial amounts of particulate matter into the lungs. It is also called occupational pneumonia.

6. **anthracosis** _____

A common type of pneumoconiosis, also called "black lung."

7. **asbestosis** _____

A common type of pneumoconiosis due to the inhalation of asbestos fibers.

8. **berylliosis** _____

A common type of pneumoconiosis due to beryllium dust.

9. **silicosis** _____

A common type of pneumoconiosis due to sand particles.

II. **SPELLING.**
   Determine if the following words are spelled correctly. If the spelling is correct, leave the word as it has already been entered. If the spelling is incorrect, provide the correct spelling.

   1. asbestosis _____   2. sereous _____

   3. sanguinous _____   4. berryliosis _____

   5. silicosis _____

III. MULTIPLE CHOICE.
Choose the best answer.

1. Occupational pneumonia.
   - ○ pneumonoconiosis
   - ○ pneumioconiosis
   - ○ pneumocionosis
   - ○ pneumoconiosis

2. Fluid containing serum and blood.
   - ○ serosanguineous
   - ○ serosanguinous
   - ○ serosanginious
   - ○ serrosanguineous

3. Inflammation of the pleura.
   - ○ pluerisy
   - ○ plueresy
   - ○ pleurisy
   - ○ plurisy

4. "Black lung."
   - ○ antharcosis
   - ○ anthracosis
   - ○ anatharcosis
   - ○ anthracoisus

5. Fluid which is clear and yellow.
   - ○ serious
   - ○ serus
   - ○ serrous
   - ○ serous

Common Respiratory Problems – Lesson 5

I. **TERMINOLOGY.**
   Enter each term in the space provided. Read the definition and description for each term.

1. **pneumonia** _____

Also called pneumonitis, this is inflammation of the lung resulting in consolidation, which is defined as a pathologic process where normally aerated lung tissue is converted into a dense, airless mass. There are many kinds of pneumonia caused by a variety of factors, the most common being a type of bacteria. It often results in hospitalization.

2. **pneumonitis** _____

Another name for pneumonia. (Pneumonia can also be viral or fungal in nature. A few of the bacterial pathogens are listed below.)

3. **consolidation** _____

A pathologic process where normally aerated lung tissue is converted into a dense, airless mass.

4. **Hemophilus influenzae** _____

This is the second most common cause of bacterial pneumonia. The most serious strain of this is type b, which is usually called Hib pneumonia.

5. **Klebsiella pneumoniae** _____

This is the most frequent of the gram-negative bacilli and it normally affects already compromised lungs, such as with the very young or the very old, hospital or nursing home patients, immuno-compromised hosts, or alcoholics.

6. **Pseudomonas aeruginosa** _____

A gram-negative pathogen.

7. **Acinetobacter** _____

A gram-negative pathogen.

8. **Legionella pneumophila** _____

Also known as Legionnaires' disease, this only accounts for 1% to 8% of pneumonias. It can occur at any age, and early phase symptoms include headache, malaise, fever, myalgia, and a cough which eventually produces mucoid sputum.

9. **Legionnaires' disease** _____

Another name for Legionella pneumophila.

10. **Mycoplasma pneumoniae** _____

This is the most common pathogen for children and young adults (age 5 to 35 years), but is otherwise quite rare. It has a long incubation period (10–14 days), which accounts for its steady spread. Early symptoms also mimic the flu, malaise, dry cough, and sore throat.

11. **Pneumococcus pneumoniae** _____

Pneumococcus pneumoniae is the most common cause for bacterial pneumonia. It usually begins with an upper respiratory infection, including congestion. The onset is often a single shaking chill followed by fever, pain with breathing, cough, dyspnea, and sputum production.

II. MULTIPLE CHOICE.
Choose the best answer.

1. A gram-negative bacilli.
   - ◯ Pseudomonis aeruginosa
   - ◯ Pseudomonas areuginosa
   - ◯ Pseudomonas aeruginosa
   - ◯ Pseudomonas aerigunosa

2. When normal lung tissue is converted into a dense, airless mass.
   - ◯ consolidation
   - ◯ consollodation
   - ◯ consolation
   - ◯ consoldation

3. The most common cause for bacterial pneumonia.
   - ◯ Pneumococus pnuemoniae
   - ◯ pneumococus pneumonniae
   - ◯ Pneumococcus Pneumoniae
   - ◯ Pneumococcus pneumoniae

4. The most frequently occurring gram-negative bacilli.
   - ◯ Klebsella pneumoniae
   - ◯ Klebsiela pneumoniae
   - ◯ klebsiella pneumoniae
   - ◯ Klebsiella pneumoniae

5. Another name for Legionella pneumophila.
   - ◯ Legionaires' disease
   - ◯ Legionnares' disease
   - ◯ Legionnaires' disease
   - ◯ Legonnaires' disease

III. MATCHING.
Match the correct term to the definition.

1. ____ Another name for pneumonia.

2. ____ A gram-negative bacilli pathogen.

3. ____ The second most common cause of bacterial pneumonia.

4. ____ Only accounts for 1% to 8% of pneumonias.

5. ____ The most common pathogen for children and young adults (age 5 to 35 years), but is otherwise quite rare.

A. pneumonitis

B. Hemophilus influenzae

C. Mycoplasma pneumoniae

D. Acinetobacter

E. Legionella pneumophila

Common Respiratory Problems – Lesson 6

I. TERMINOLOGY.
Enter each term in the space provided. Read the definition and description for each term.

1. Staphylococcus aureus _____

Staphylococcus aureus accounts for approximately 2% of community-acquired pneumonias. Patients at particular risk are infants, the elderly, hospitalized patients, surgical patients, and patients with immunosuppression. Its symptoms closely mimic those of pneumococcal pneumoniae, although the mortality rate is as high as 30% to 40%.

2. Streptococcus pneumoniae _____

This has become relatively rare since World War I and is usually a complication of influenza, measles, chickenpox, or pertussis.

3. pneumothorax _____

Free air in the pleural cavity between the visceral and parietal pleurae. It may occur either spontaneously or because of trauma or pathological process.

4. rhinitis _____

Inflammation of the mucous membranes of the nose. Often accompanied by rhinorrhea (a runny nose).

5. rhinorrhea _____

Runny nose.

6. sarcoidosis _____

Also called Boeck sarcoid, this is a systemic disease of unknown etiology with the most severe manifestation being granulomatous pneumonitis.

7. Boeck sarcoid _____

Another name for sarcoidosis.

8. **granulomatous** _____

Pertaining to any small nodular aggregation of a certain kind of cells.

9. **sinusitis** _____

Inflammation of a sinus. It is usually designated by the name of the sinus that is inflamed (e.g., ethmoid sinusitis).

10. **tonsillitis** _____

Inflammation of the tonsils, especially the palatine tonsils.

II. **SPELLING.**
   Determine if the following words are spelled correctly. If the spelling is correct, leave the word as it has already been entered. If the spelling is incorrect, provide the correct spelling.

1. rrhinorhea _____   2. Boeck sarcoid _____

3. Streptococus pneumoniae _____   4. tonsilitis _____

5. sarcodoisis _____

III. **MULTIPLE CHOICE.**
   Choose the best answer.

1. The bacteria (⃝staphylococcus areus, ⃝Staphylococcus aureus) causes pneumonia with a high mortality rate.

2. Free air in the pleural cavity is referred to as a (⃝pneumothorax, ⃝pneumothroax) .

3. Inflammation of the mucous membranes is called ((⃝rhinitis, ⃝rhinoitis) .

4. Inflammation of the sinus is (⃝sinusitis, ⃝sinisitis)

5. The most severe pneumonitis is called (⃝granulomatous, ⃝granualomatous) .

233

Common Respiratory Problems – Lesson 7

I. TERMINOLOGY.
   Enter each term in the space provided. Read the definition and description for each term.

   1. **tracheitis** _____

   Inflammation of the trachea.

   2. **tuberculosis** _____

   A chronic, recurrent infection most common in the lungs, although any organ may be affected. Once infection is established (via a PPD skin test and sputum culture), symptoms may develop within months or may be dormant for many years. It specifically refers to a disease caused by Mycobacterium tuberculosis. Active pulmonary TB has a great potential to destroy lung and to kill, but is often asymptomatic except for "not feeling well." Cough, dyspnea, and pleural effusion usually progress over the course of the disease. The most famous symptom, hemoptysis, is usually not seen in the early stages. TB is potentially highly infectious.

   3. **Mycobacterium tuberculosis** _____

   The gram-positive bacterium that causes tuberculosis.

   4. **upper respiratory infection (URI)** _____

   The common cold. An acute, usually afebrile viral infection of the respiratory tract with inflammation in any or all of the airways, including the nose, paranasal sinuses, throat, larynx, and often the trachea and bronchi. You are probably familiar with the symptoms.

   5. **Wegener's granulomatosis** _____

   An uncommon disease that usually begins as a localized granulomatous inflammation of the upper and/or lower respiratory tract mucosa.

II. SPELLING.
   Determine if the following words are spelled correctly. If the spelling is correct, leave the word as it has already been entered. If the spelling is incorrect, provide the correct spelling.

   1. Myocobacterium _____   2. Wegener's granulomatosis _____

   3. trachiitis _____   4. tuberculosus _____

   5. granulomatosis _____

III. MULTIPLE CHOICE.
Choose the best answer.

1. Inflammation of the trachea.
   - ◯ traceitis
   - ◯ tracheitis
   - ◯ trachitis
   - ◯ tracheoitis

2. The bacterium responsible for tuberculosis.
   - ◯ mycobacterium tuberculosis
   - ◯ Mycobacterium tuberculosis
   - ◯ micobacterium tuberculosis
   - ◯ Mycobacterum tuberculosis

3. Disease of the respiratory tract mucosa.
   - ◯ Wegner's granulomatosis
   - ◯ Wegener's granulomatous
   - ◯ Wegener's granulomatosis
   - ◯ Wagener's granulomatosis

4. The common cold.
   - ◯ uper respiratory infection
   - ◯ upper respirratory infection
   - ◯ upper respiriatory infection
   - ◯ upper respiratory infection

5. A chronic, recurrent infection most common in the lungs, although any organ may be affected.
   - ◯ tubercelosis
   - ◯ tubercelosus
   - ◯ tuberculosis
   - ◯ tuberculosus

Something to Remember

By now you should have a better understanding of what is involved with the process of respiration and how it can affect your health.

Pneumonia, for example, is quite common in a hospital setting and therefore any acute care work that you deal with will include admissions, discharges, x-rays, and therapy related to this problem.

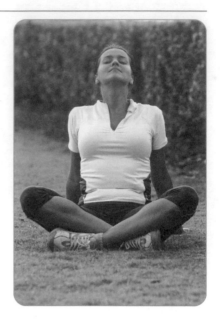

It is noteworthy that pneumonia is also a serious potential risk of any hospital stay, as it is one of the most common nosocomial infections. A nosocomial infection is one that is acquired in the hospital setting. In other words, it refers to some pathology that was not present in a patient upon admission to the hospital but that occurs approximately 72 hours after admission.

Additionally, because of the impact of colds and flu upon the respiratory system, the terminology found in this unit is utilized commonly in clinic and doctor's office settings.

Unit 7
Reproductive System

Reproductive System – Introduction

The reproductive system is not vital to the function and health of the human body, but it exists to perpetuate the species and pass genetic material from one generation to another. Most of the smallest details of human reproduction occur cyclically within the human male and female and are not, therefore, significant to the function of the body as a whole.

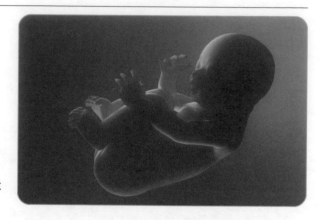

An incredible amount of information is currently available on the process of human reproduction. Because of this knowledge, laboratories in clinics and hospitals throughout the world are able to recreate many of the natural reproductive functions on behalf of couples who struggle with infertility.

The focus of this unit will be on understanding the basic structure of both sexes and the potentiality for disease and not on the overall process of reproduction. Additionally, this unit will contain information on the urinary or excretory system. The urinary system is closely related to the reproductive system in that they are anatomically close and even share certain organs, especially in the male.

It is necessary for male and female anatomy, as they relate to the reproductive system, to be studied separately. The first part of this unit will discuss the female reproductive system. This includes the parts necessary to both create and sustain life prior to and following birth, including the nourishment of a newborn child.

Female Reproductive System

The structures of the female reproductive system can be grouped based on their location in the body into either the internal organs of reproduction or the external genitalia. These organs are responsible for the induction of menstruation and for the hosting and development of the sexual components that create fetuses and for the fetuses themselves.

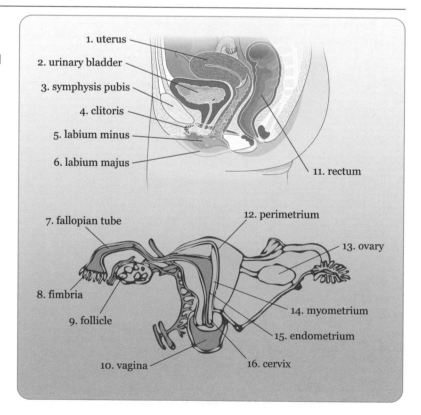

1. uterus
2. urinary bladder
3. symphysis pubis
4. clitoris
5. labium minus
6. labium majus
7. fallopian tube
8. fimbria
9. follicle
10. vagina
11. rectum
12. perimetrium
13. ovary
14. myometrium
15. endometrium
16. cervix

I. FILL IN THE BLANK.

In the blanks provided below, refer to the image and enter the term corresponding to the following numbers. Use the word(s) in the box to fill in the blanks.

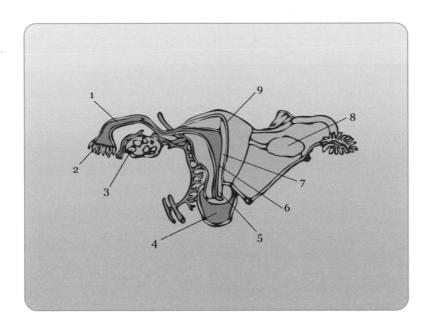

1. _____

2. _____

3. _____

4. _____

5. _____

6. _____

7. _____

8. _____

9. _____

| myometrium |
| vagina |
| perimetrium |
| fimbria |
| fallopian tube |
| ovary |
| cervix |
| follicle |
| endometrium |

II. FILL IN THE BLANK.

In the blanks provided below, refer to the image and enter the term corresponding to the following numbers. Use the word(s) in the box to fill in the blanks.

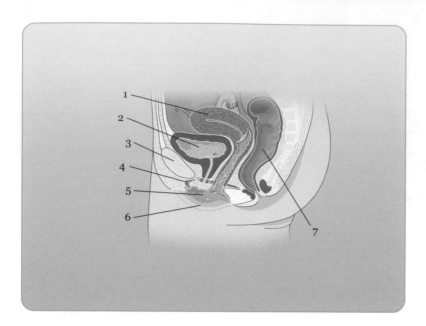

1. _____

2. _____

3. _____

4. _____

5. _____

6. _____

7. _____

clitoris
urinary bladder
rectum
uterus
labium majus
symphysis pubis
labium minus

Internal Female Organs

The female has four primary sex organs: ovaries, fallopian tubes, uterus, and vagina. The ovaries are paired organs that not only produce gametes (ova or eggs), they are also responsible for the production of the two female hormones: estrogen and progesterone. Ovaries are oval in shape and measure approximately 3.5 cm long, 2 cm wide, and 1 cm thick. Positioned on either side of the uterus, the ovaries are supported by a mesentery that consists of the mesovarium, suspensory, and ovarian ligaments. Each ovary has an outer cortex and an inner medulla. The connective tissue of the cortex is called its stroma, and throughout the stroma are many ovarian follicles in various stages of development.

Reproductive Process

Ovaries produce eggs

Egg released into fallopian tube

Egg transported to uterus

Egg is fertilized or not fertilized

Fertilized egg attaches to uterine wall

Normally only one ovarian follicle develops or matures each month. During maturation, the follicle enlarges and develops a second layer, the cells of which produce the female hormone, estrogen. This mature follicle measures approximately 1 cm in diameter and is called a graafian follicle. During ovulation, the surface of the follicles gives way and allows the ovum to escape. The ruptured follicle then develops into a corpus luteum. The cells that make up its lining enlarge and develop yellow granules, which are the source for the other female hormone, progesterone.

Once the ovum is released, it enters the open end of the fallopian tube nearest to it. The fallopian tubes (also called uterine tubes or oviducts) transport the ovum to the uterus. Each fallopian tube is narrow, smooth, and muscular and measures approximately 10 cm in length. The lumen of each tube is lined with cilia and epithelial cells. The narrow isthmus of each tube opens directly into the uterus. The longest portion of the tube is called the ampulla and the funnel-shaped distal end is the infundibulum.

After it leaves the uterine tube, the ovum enters the uterus—a hollow, thick-walled, muscular organ that is shaped somewhat like an inverted pear. Positioned between the urinary bladder and the rectum, the uterus is not firmly attached and can be tilted as necessary (for example, when the bladder is full). The main portion of the uterus is called the body; the tapered distal portion is the cervix; and the uppermost portion is referred to as the fundus. The wall of the uterus is composed of three layers. The inner lining, or endometrium, undergoes changes based on the menstrual cycle. After each period, there is a proliferative stage in which the endometrium rapidly regenerates and the blood supply increases. In the secretory stage the endometrium develops further and the glands become large and coiled. At this point, the endometrium is ready for a fertilized embryo. If this does not occur, the menstrual stage follows, during which the built-up endometrium quickly breaks down and sloughs away, revealing the thin layer underneath—the myometrium. Because the prefix my/o means muscle, it's easy to remember this layer is composed of smooth muscle. The outermost layer of the uterus is the perimetrium, a membranous lining that secretes serous fluid.

The vagina is a muscular tube about 9.5 cm in length that passes from the cervical opening, or os, to the uterus and to the outside of the body. A recessed area around the cervix, the fornix, functions as both a receptacle for a penis during sexual intercourse (and repository for sperm) and as the birth canal for parturition (the birthing process). It becomes lubricated during sexual excitement by secretions from the vestibular or Bartholin's glands, as well as by secretions from the mucous glands of the cervix.

I. TERMINOLOGY.
Enter each term in the space provided. Read the definition and description for each term.

1. **ovaries** _____
Paired organs that produce gametes and the hormones estrogen and progesterone.

2. **fallopian tubes** _____
Tubes that transport the ovum to the uterus.

3. **uterus** _____
A hollow muscular organ where the fetus matures.

4. **vagina** _____
A muscular tube that passes from the cervical opening to the uterus and to the outside of the body.

5. **ampulla** _____
The longest portion of the fallopian tube.

6. **infundibulum** _____
The funnel-shaped distal end of the fallopian tube.

7. **cervix** _____
The tapered distal portion of the uterus.

8. **endometrium** _____
The inner lining of the uterus that undergoes changes based on the menstrual cycle.

II. MULTIPLE CHOICE.
Choose the best answer.

1. What is the thin under-layer of the uterus called?
   - ○ myometrium
   - ○ enometrium
   - ○ cervix
   - ○ fornix

2. The endometrium is ready for a fertilized embryo at which stage?
   - ○ the proliferative stage when the blood supply increases
   - ○ the secretory stage when the glands become large and coiled
   - ○ the menstrual stage when the endometrium breaks down and sloughs away
   - ○ the final stage when the endometrium is fully sloughed away

3. How many ovarian follicles usually develop or mature each month?

    ○ 1
    ○ 2
    ○ 3
    ○ 4

4. The area that serves as the birth canal is called the _____.

    ○ fundus
    ○ cervix
    ○ fornix
    ○ corpus luteum

External Female Organs

The other organs of the female reproductive system are the external genitalia, also called the vulva. The vulva consists of the mons pubis, a pad of connective tissue that covers the symphysis pubis and (after puberty) supports the coarse pubic hair. The labia majora (plural) are two longitudinal folds of skin comprised of adipose and muscular tissue. They are continuous with the mons pubis and eventually form the perineum (the area between the thighs to the anus). The labia majora are covered with hair and contain multiple sebaceous glands, which secrete a greasy, lubricating substance.

1. fatty tissue

2. milk ducts

3. areola

4. nipple

5. lobules

The labia minora (plural) are two smaller longitudinal folds located between the labia majora. They are hairless, contain sebaceous glands, and split to form the prepuce (fold of skin) that covers the clitoris. The clitoris, a small rounded structure made up of erectile tissue and sensitive epithelium, is found at the upper portion of the vestibule (the cleft between the labia into which both the vagina and urethra open).

You may remember from your study of the skeletal system that the pelvis includes the hip bones, the pubic bones, and the symphysis pubis, the fibrocartilaginous joint formed by the junction of the pubic bones.

And finally, also included in the female reproductive system are the mammary glands. Structurally, these glands within the breasts are modified sweat glands and are actually a part of the integumentary (skin) system. Functionally, however, they are associated with the reproductive system because they secrete milk for nourishment of infants (a process called lactation). Each gland is composed of 15 to 20 lobes with a duct that opens at the tip of the nipple. The nipple itself is partially composed of erectile tissue and is surrounded by a circular area, the areola, that is usually darker in pigment than the surrounding skin.

I. **TRUE/FALSE.**
   Mark the following true or false.

   1. The labia minora support coarse pubic hair after puberty.

      ○ true
      ○ false

   2. The clitoris is a small, rounded structure made up of erectile tissue and epithelium.

      ○ true
      ○ false

   3. The mons pubis is a pad of connective tissue that covers the symphysis pubis.

      ○ true
      ○ false

   4. The labia majora contain sebaceous glands which secrete a greasy, lubricating substance.

      ○ true
      ○ false

   5. The vulva is the area between the thighs to the anus.

      ○ true
      ○ false

II. FILL IN THE BLANK.
In the blanks provided below, refer to the above image and enter the term corresponding to the following numbers. Use the word(s) in the box to fill in the blanks.

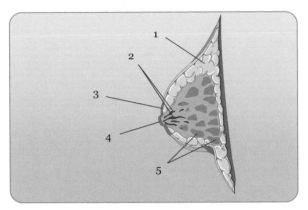

1. _____

2. _____

3. _____

4. _____

5. _____

nipple
lobules
fatty tissue
areola
milk ducts

Female Reproductive Anatomy – Lesson 1

I. TERMINOLOGY.
Enter each term in the space provided. Read the definition and description for each term.

1. **eggs** _____

Gametes or ova.

2. **estrogen** _____

A female hormone secreted by the ovary, it is responsible for typical female sexual characteristics.

3. **progesterone** _____

A female hormone that prepares and maintains the uterus for pregnancy.

4. **mesentery** _____

A double layer of peritoneum that acts as a structural support for the ovaries.

5. **mesovarium** _____

The fold of peritoneum connecting the ovary with the wall of the abdominal cavity.

6. **suspensory ligament** _____

A fold of peritoneum that extends out from the ovary to the wall of the pelvis. (Also called infundibulopelvic ligament.)

7. **ovarian ligament** _____

A fibrous ligament that connects the ovary to the lateral surface of the uterus. (Also called utero-ovarian ligament.)

8. **cortex** _____

Outer portion of an organ.

9. **medulla** _____

Inner part of an organ.

10. **stroma** _____

The connective tissue of the cortex that contains many ovarian follicles in various stages of development.

11. **graafian follicle** _____

Matured ovarian follicle that produces the female hormone estrogen.

12. **corpus luteum** _____

The ruptured ovarian follicle that produces the female hormone progesterone.

13. **oviducts** _____

Another name for the fallopian tubes.

14. **ampulla** _____

The longest portion of the fallopian tube.

15. **infundibulum** _____

The widest end of the fallopian tube; it is funnel shaped.

Female Reproductive Anatomy – Lesson 2

I. **TERMINOLOGY.**
   Enter each term in the space provided. Read the definition and description for each term.

   1. **fundus** _____

   The upper most portion of the uterus.

   2. **proliferative** _____

   A stage in the menstrual cycle where the endometrium rapidly regenerates and the blood supply increases.

3. **fornix** _____

A recessed area around the cervix.

4. **vestibular** _____

Lubricating glands for the fornix.

5. **Bartholin's gland** _____

Lubricating glands for the fornix.

6. **vulva** _____

Part of the female reproductive system called the external genitalia.

7. **mons pubis** _____

A pad of connective tissue that covers the symphysis pubis and (after puberty) supports the coarse pubic hair.

8. **perineum** _____

The area between the thighs to the anus.

9. **sebaceous glands** _____

Glands which secrete a greasy, lubricating substance.

10. **prepuce** _____

A covering fold of skin of the clitoris.

11. **mammary** _____

Glands located within the breasts that are modified sweat glands.

12. **integumentary** _____

The skin.

13. **lactation** _____

The secretion of milk from the breasts for nourishment of infants.

14. **areola** _____

A circular pigmented area that surrounds the nipple.

Review: Female Reproduction

I. **MULTIPLE CHOICE.**
   Choose the best answer.

1. A mature follicle.
   - ○ mons pubis
   - ○ estrogen
   - ○ graafian follicle
   - ○ progesterone

2. A pad of connective tissue covering the symphysis pubis.
   - ○ perineum
   - ○ mons pubis
   - ○ oviducts
   - ○ gametes

3. The reproductive system can be divided into the internal organs and the _____.
   - ○ mons pubis
   - ○ internal genitalia
   - ○ external genitalia
   - ○ perineum

4. A covering fold of skin.
   - ○ prepuce
   - ○ follicle
   - ○ mesentery
   - ○ cortex

5. The distal end of the uterine tube.
   - ○ areola
   - ○ perineum
   - ○ ova
   - ○ infundibulum

6. A circular pigmented area.
   - ○ areola
   - ○ pubis
   - ○ ampulla
   - ○ vestibular

7. The longest portion of the fallopian tube.
   - ◯ Bartholin's gland
   - ◯ vulva
   - ◯ ampulla
   - ◯ areola

8. The connective tissue of the cortex.
   - ◯ stroma
   - ◯ sebaceous
   - ◯ mesentery
   - ◯ vulva

9. The uppermost portion of the uterus.
   - ◯ stroma
   - ◯ corpus luteum
   - ◯ oviducts
   - ◯ fundus

10. Another term for the external genitalia.
    - ◯ ova
    - ◯ vulva
    - ◯ gametes
    - ◯ lactation

11. The ovaries are located on either side of the uterus and are supported by this.
    - ◯ menses
    - ◯ perineum
    - ◯ mesentery
    - ◯ medulla

12. A gland that lubricates the vagina during sexual excitement.
    - ◯ Bartholin gland
    - ◯ secretory phase
    - ◯ fornix
    - ◯ cortex

13. The first of the female hormones.
    - ◯ progesterone
    - ◯ estrogen
    - ◯ stroma
    - ◯ ova

14. Glands that secrete a greasy substance.

○ lactation
○ menses
○ sebaceous
○ mesovarium

15. A ligament that comprises the mesentery.

○ mesovarium
○ gametes or ova
○ oviducts
○ fornix

16. The inner portion of an ovary.

○ prepuce
○ areola
○ mons pubis
○ medulla

17. The ruptured follicle that generates progesterone.

○ mesovarium
○ fornix
○ corpus luteum
○ menses

18. The area between the thighs.

○ vulva
○ symphysis pubis
○ perineum
○ cortex

19. The cyclic discharge of blood and tissues from the uterus.

○ menstruation
○ mons pubis
○ secretory phase
○ ampulla

20. Another name for #19.

○ menses
○ lactation
○ secretory phase
○ mesovarium

21. The secretion of milk.

○ menses
○ lactation
○ milk ducts
○ secretory phase

22. Modified sweat glands.

○ sebaceous glands
○ Bartholin's glands
○ mammary glands
○ vestibular glands

23. The outer surface of an ovary.

○ cortex
○ fornix
○ medulla
○ follicle

24. The recessed area around the cervix.

○ prepuce
○ vortex
○ fornix
○ mons pubis

25. Another term for fallopian tubes.

○ mammary glands
○ oviducts
○ tubal ligation
○ mesovarium

26. The joint formed by a union of the pubic bones by thick fibrocartilage.

○ mons pubis
○ mesentery
○ secretory phase
○ symphysis pubis

27. The middle stage through which the uterine lining progresses.

○ secretory phase

○ lactation

○ menses

○ oviducts

28. The main product of the ovaries.

○ areola

○ gametes or ova

○ estrogen

○ progesterone

Female Reproductive System Specialty (OB/GYN)

The diagnosis and treatment of problems associated with pregnancy and the female reproductive system are carried out in obstetrics and gynecology departments. The physician who treats female problems is a gynecologist, and the doctor who delivers babies is an obstetrician. Generally, a physician specializes in both areas, and the abbreviation for the doctor and the department is OB/GYN.

A good portion of OB/GYN, logically, is dedicated to the prevention, assistance, or progress of pregnancy. OB/GYN and family practice physicians discuss these options with patients and offer advice on using them.

There are many options available to prevent pregnancy from occurring, including birth control pills, long-acting birth control shots, IUDs (intrauterine devices), sponges, diaphragms, implants, and others. Surgical procedures, such as vasectomy or tubal ligation, are more permanent options for birth control. Vasectomy is a procedure performed on men to prevent sperm from being transferred during sexual intercourse. It is an outpatient procedure and is performed quite frequently. A similar procedure performed on women is a tubal ligation in which the uterine tubes are either cut or ligated (tied). This procedure is generally irreversible; however, in some cases microsurgery can be performed to reopen or reattach the uterine tubes.

Assessing Female Reproductive System

In medicine, the establishment or beginning of menstrual function is called menarche. The cessation of menstruation, generally occurring at approximately age 50, is called menopause. Once menstruation has started, regular examinations with a gynecologist should begin. These are annual examinations during which the overall health of the reproductive system is ascertained. Standard during this examination is a Pap smear.

This is an acceptable shortened form for Papanicolaou smear. The Pap test examines the cells of the female tract (cervix, endometrium, and vagina) to determine if there are any precancerous or cancerous lesions. The annual exam also includes regular breast examinations to palpate lumps, and eventually (after age 35) mammograms are ordered to examine the breasts radiographically for lesions. A bimanual examination is also standard, and literally means an examination with both hands. In gynecology, one hand (or fingers only) is placed in the vagina and the other on the abdomen, in order to palpate the uterus.

The Department of Health and Human Resources recommends women have Pap smears as part of their routine health maintenance, as an average of 3700 women die of cervical cancer each year.

Why do I need a Pap test?

A Pap test can save your life. It can find the earliest signs of cervical cancer—a common cancer in women. If caught early, the chance of curing cervical cancer is very high. Pap tests also can find infections and abnormal cervical cells that can turn into cancer cells. Treatment can prevent most cases of cervical cancer from developing.

Getting regular Pap tests is the best thing you can do to prevent cervical cancer. About 13,000 women in America will find out they have cervical cancer this year.*

(U.S. Department of Health and Human Services. www.4women.gov/faq/pap-test.cfm)

If a woman desires pregnancy, certain factors need to be within normal parameters to optimize the possibility. These include the presence of estradiol (the most potent naturally-occurring estrogen in humans) and FSH (follicle-stimulating hormone secreted by the hypothalamus to enable follicles to develop properly). The levels of these two hormones are determined with a blood test. It is also necessary that the luteal phase, which is the number of days between ovulation and the last day of the menstrual cycle, be long enough for pregnancy to occur. (This is named for the corpus luteum and is also called the postovulatory phase).

Finally, the internal organs of the reproductive system need to be present and functioning properly (i.e., not blocked or otherwise damaged). The state of the internal organs can be assessed through various means. Common procedures include ultrasounds, hysterosalpingograms (a dye-test with visualization of the tubes and uterus by x-ray), and laparoscopies (examination of the interior of the abdomen or pelvis with a scope) with chromotubation (a dye-test of the tubes under direct or camera visualization).

I. FILL IN THE BLANK.
Using the word/word parts in the box, fill in the blanks.

hysterosalpingogram
menarche
Pap smear
luteal phase
bimanual examination
estradiol

1. The shortened name for the test that examines the cells of the female tract for any precancerous or cancerous lesions is called a _____.

2. The _____ is the number of days between ovulation and the last day of the menstrual cycle.

3. The establishment or beginning of menstrual function is called _____.

4. A standard examination called a _____ means an examination with both hands.

5. A dye-test with visualization of the tubes and uterus by x-ray is called a _____.

6. For pregnancy to occur, the hormones _____ and FSH must be present.

Pregnancy

Assuming that everything is working okay, pregnancy is possible. In order to determine if a woman is pregnant, a standard pregnancy test is performed. This test assesses the presence of HCG (human chorionic gonadotropin) in either the blood or the urine. If HCG is present, the woman is pregnant.

In humans, the normal gestation period is 40 weeks—the time from the first day of the mother's last menstrual cycle through birth. A pregnant woman is described as being a gravida (pregnant woman) because she has a gravid (pregnant) uterus. Gravidity increases with each pregnancy. Therefore, a woman who has been pregnant twice is gravida 2. Parity describes the outcome of each pregnancy and is described in two ways. Each delivery after 20 weeks is considered a para (1, 2, 3, etc.). Each loss, whether voluntary or spontaneous, is an abortus (1, 2, 3, etc.). This is sometimes designated as AB (1, 2, 3, etc.). Occasionally, a fourth number is assigned to designate the number of living children.

Once pregnancy is established, it is recommended that a woman visit her obstetrician monthly for prenatal care. Aside from routine ultrasounds that determine normal fetal development, there are other tests that many pregnant women choose to have performed. The first, done at approximately 16 weeks' gestation, is the maternal serum alpha fetoprotein (MSAFP). Elevated levels can indicate neural tube defect, multiple fetuses, or incorrect dates. Low levels indicate some chromosomal abnormalities (such as Down's syndrome). An amniocentesis is commonly performed at approximately 15 to 17 weeks gestation. This is a needle aspiration of the uterus to obtain amniotic fluid for determination of abnormalities.

Highlights

A pregnant woman is described as gravida (G). The outcome of pregnancy is known as parity. Parity is designated by either a (P) for para or an (AB) for abortus. A woman who is pregnant and has had two miscarriages and three living children would be designated G6, P3, AB2, 3.

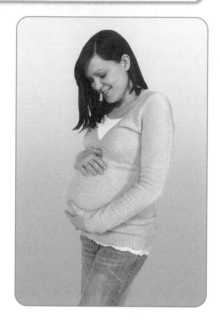

I. MATCHING.
Match the correct term to the definition.

1. ____ HCG
2. ____ gravida
3. ____ parity
4. ____ AB
5. ____ MSAFP

A. pregnant woman
B. pregnancy outcome
C. a test indicating defects and chromosomal abnormalities
D. indicates voluntary or spontaneous loss
E. the hormone that indicates pregnancy in the blood or urine

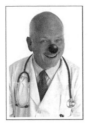

Pregnancy Humor

Q: When will my baby move?
A: With any luck, right after high school.

Q: What is the most common pregnancy craving?
A: For men to be the ones who get pregnant.

Q. What is the most reliable method to determine a baby's sex?
A: Childbirth.

Childbirth

At approximately 40 weeks' gestation, the child should be ready to be born. There are several things that happen prior to and during this event. Most of the following states are determined upon examination by a physician or midwife. To begin, the baby "drops," which is a move in the uterus to the birth canal; this can happen at any time in the last month before delivery. It is necessary for the fetus to descend as this starts the changes in the female body to allow passage of the fetus. The level of the fetus in the pelvic cavity is referred to as the "station." This is designated by +1, 0, -1, etc.

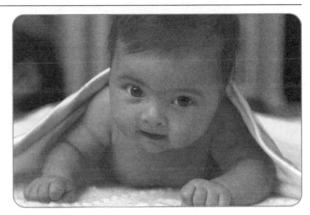

Prior to delivery, a mucus plug is released, and the bag of waters (amniotic sac) ruptures. If the physician does this it is called an amniotomy; otherwise it is the spontaneous rupture of membranes.

The presentation is the position of the lowermost part of the fetus, such as breech (buttocks), vertex (the crown of the head), or shoulder.

A vertex presentation is optimal. The degree of effacement and dilation of the cervix are also determined.

Effacement is the obliteration and change of the cervix that occurs during labor, so that only the thin external os remains. (Os is simply a term for an orifice.)

Dilation of the cervix is recorded in centimeters according to the width of the diameter of the cervix.

If a delivery is accomplished vaginally, it is considered a "normal" delivery. This can be assisted medically with a variety of instruments and procedures, including an episiotomy (surgical incision into the perineum and vagina), internal and external fetal monitors, forceps (an instrument with two blades and a handle for grasping tissues, in this case, the baby's head), suction or vacuum extraction, and a variety of drugs and synthetic hormones to stimulate, regulate, and expedite labor.

Following delivery of the baby is the delivery of the placenta. This is the organ through which blood, nutrients, and fluids are shared between the mother and the fetus, and how waste is removed.

Also following delivery, the newborn infant has an Apgar score assessment. The assessment is a numerical expression (0–10) of the condition of the newborn based on such factors as the respiratory rate, heart rate, muscle tone, reflex to stimulation, and color. It is usually assessed at both one minute and five minutes after birth.

The child is also weighed and measured.

The period for the mother after childbirth is called the postpartum period. This designates the period immediately following childbirth to four weeks after delivery.

Following parturition there is a vaginal discharge during the first one to two weeks, or sometimes longer, which is called lochia. A number of other terms are associated with the process of conception (or preventing it), pregnancy, delivery, and the postpartum period. The above is a broad outline of these complex processes.

I. **MULTIPLE CHOICE.**
    Choose the best answer.

1. A baby who presents with buttocks first as called (○vertex, ○breech) .

2. Vaginal discharge during the first 1 to 2 weeks after parturition is called (○lochia, ○mucus plug) .

3. (○effacement, ○dilation) is the obliteration and change of the cervix that occurs during labor.

4. A physician performs an (○amniotomy, ○spontaneous rupture of membranes) to rupture the amniotic sac.

5. A surgical incision into the perineum and vagina, or (○effacement, ○episiotomy) is a medical procedure to assist in vaginal delivery.

6. The level of the fetus in the pelvic cavity is referred to as the (○drop, ○station) .

7. The numerical assessment of a newborn's condition is called an (○Apgar, ○Apnea) score assessment.

8. The organ through which blood, nutrients, and fluids are shared between the mother and the fetus is called the (○uterus, ○placenta) .

9. The period following childbirth for the mother is known as the (○postpartum, ○lochia) period.

10. The dilation of the cervix is recorded in (○centimeters, ○inches) .

Female Reproductive Terminology – Lesson 1

I. **TERMINOLOGY.**
   Enter each term in the space provided. Read the definition and description for each term.

1. **puberty** _____

   The time when secondary sex changes begin.

2. **menarche** _____

   The establishment or beginning of menstrual function.

3. **menopause** _____

   Cessation of menstruation, generally occurring at approximately age 50.

4. **Papanicolaou smear** _____

   This test examines the cells of the female tract (cervix, endometrium, and vagina) to determine if there are any precancerous or cancerous lesions.

5. **mammograms** _____

   Radiographs of the breasts to check for lesions.

6. **bimanual** _____

   An examination with both hands; one hand (or fingers only) is placed in the vagina and the other on the abdomen, in order to palpate the uterus.

7. **estradiol** _____

   The most potent naturally-occurring estrogen in humans.

8. **FSH** _____

   Follicle-stimulating hormone secreted by the hypothalamus that enables follicles to develop properly.

9. **luteal phase** _____

   Named for the corpus luteum and is also known as the postovulatory phase.

10. **hysterosalpingogram** _____

   A dye-test with visualization of the tubes and uterus by x-ray(fluoroscopy).

11. **laparoscopy** _____

   Examination of the interior of the abdomen or pelvis with a scope.

12. **chromotubation** _____

   A dye-test of the tubes under direct or camera visualization.

13. **human chorionic gonadotropin** _____

   Hormone present in the blood that indicates pregnancy.

14. **gestation** _____

   The time from the first day of the mother's last menstrual cycle through birth.

15. **gravida** _____

A pregnant woman. Often used in conjunction with a number to notate the number of pregnancies a woman has had.

16. **parity** _____

The outcome of each pregnancy.

17. **para** _____

Each delivery of a fetus after 20 weeks of gestation.

Female Reproductive Terminology – Lesson 2

I. **TERMINOLOGY.**
   Enter each term in the space provided. Read the definition and description for each term.

1. **abortus** _____

Each loss of a fetus.

2. **maternal serum alpha-fetoprotein** _____

A blood test to check levels of alpha-fetoprotein, which, if elevated, can indicate neural tube defect, multiple fetuses, or incorrect dates.

3. **amniocentesis** _____

A needle aspiration of the uterus to obtain amniotic fluid for determination of abnormalities.

4. **amniotomy** _____

The delivery of a mucous plug and rupture of the bag of waters (amniotic sac) performed by the physician.

5. **breech** _____

Presentation of the infant buttocks first.

6. **vertex** _____

Presentation of the infant with the crown of the head/shoulder first.

7. **effacement** _____

The obliteration and change of the cervix that occurs during labor.

8. **dilation** _____

The amount of opening of the cervix during labor, measured in centimeters according to the width and diameter of the cervix.

9. **external os** _____

External orifice.

10. **episiotomy** _____

Surgical incision into the perineum and vagina.

11. **forceps** _____

An instrument with two blades and a handle for grasping the baby's head.

12. **placenta** _____

The organ through which blood, nutrients, and fluids are shared between the mother and the fetus and waste is removed.

13. **Apgar score** _____

An assessment of the newborn in a numerical expression (0–10) based on such factors as the respiratory rate, heart rate, muscle tone, reflex to stimulation, and color; usually assessed at both one minute and five minutes after birth.

14. **postpartum** _____

The period for the mother after childbirth.

15. **lochia** _____

A vaginal discharge during the first one to two weeks after childbirth.

16. **vasectomy** _____

A surgical procedure performed on men to prevent the transfer of sperm via intercourse.

17. **tubal ligation** _____

A surgical procedure performed on women to prevent pregnancy.

Female Reproductive Diseases – Lesson 1

As mentioned earlier in this unit, the function of the reproductive system is not vital to sustaining life. Reproductive organs and structures, however, can harbor infections or diseases that can threaten health and well-being. Furthermore, because of the compelling nature to propagate the species, including the "maternal instinct" that prompts women to conceive, carry, and nurture children, any problem related to this system which prevents that from happening is certainly significant—to both the woman who experiences it and to her healthcare professionals. As a result, many of these problems are defined and treated medically.

Aside from abnormal pathology that affects the reproductive system generally, there are terms that deal specifically with pregnancy. In addition, complications associated with pregnancy are routinely treated by obstetricians. As with other systems, certain symptoms can be evaluated to determine the presence of reproductive problems.

I. TERMINOLOGY.
Enter each term in the space provided. Read the definition and description for each term.

1. **amenorrhea** _____
Absence or abnormal stoppage of menstrual flow.

2. **dysmenorrhea** _____
Painful menstruation.

3. **dyspareunia** _____
Difficult or painful coitus.

4. **coitus** _____
Sexual connection of male and female; another term for intercourse.

5. **dysuria** _____
Painful or difficult urination. Although this is a symptom that affects the urinary system, it can also be indicative of reproductive pathology.

6. **hirsutism** _____
Abnormal hairiness. This refers to the condition in which a male pattern of hair distribution occurs in a woman. It comes from the root "hirsute," meaning "hairy."

7. **menometrorrhagia** _____
Excessive uterine bleeding that occurs both during menses and at irregular intervals. This is a common symptom in menopausal women.

8. **menorrhea** _____
This term is used interchangeably to mean both the normal flow of menstruation and profuse menstruation.

9. **metrorrhagia** _____
Uterine bleeding which occurs in varying amounts at totally irregular intervals, sometimes lasting for a long time.

10. **mittelschmerz** _____
Pain which occurs during ovulation (which is generally the middle of a menstrual cycle).

11. **oligomenorrhea** _____
Infrequent menstrual flow, usually occurring in cycles of 35 days to six months.

12. **pica** _____
A bizarre craving for strange foods, or even inedible materials such as dirt, gravel, paint, or plaster. This sometimes occurs in pregnant women.

13. **pruritus vulvi** _____
Severe itching of the external genitalia.

Female Reproductive Diseases – Lesson 2

I. TERMINOLOGY.
Enter each term in the space provided. Read the definition and description for each term.

1. **abortion** _____

The premature expulsion from the uterus of the products of conception—generally a nonviable fetus. There are different types of abortions. The most common that you will see in medical reports are spontaneous and therapeutic abortions. A spontaneous abortion is a naturally occurring one, often referred to in layman's terms as a miscarriage. A therapeutic abortion is one that is deliberately induced by a physician.

2. **spontaneous abortion** _____

One of the most common types of abortions seen in medical reports.

3. **miscarriage** _____

Naturally occurring abortion.

4. **therapeutic abortion** _____

Abortion deliberately induced by a physician.

5. **abruptio placentae** _____

A premature detachment of the placenta. This is usually fatal to the unborn fetus.

6. **anovulation** _____

The absence of ovulation. This can be used to describe a woman either before she begins her menstrual cycle or following menopause. There are also a variety of reasons for this to occur otherwise—such as with extreme obesity or very low body weight, stress, or drugs.

7. **Asherman syndrome** _____

Persistent amenorrhea and secondary sterility due to intrauterine adhesions.

8. **candidiasis** _____

Generically this is any infection caused by a fungus of the genus Candida. It is usually a superficial infection of moist areas of the body—and is commonly seen in the vagina.

9. **cervicitis** _____

Inflammation of the cervix.

10. **cesarean section** _____

Incision through the abdominal and uterine walls for delivery of a baby.

11. **Chlamydia** _____

A genus of bacteria that multiply only within a host cell. This is a common sexually transmitted disease and secondarily causes infertility, especially in female patients.

12. **dystocia** _____

Abnormal or difficult labor. This may be caused by obstruction or constriction of the birth passage, or by some abnormality in the size, shape, condition, or position of the fetus.

13. **endometriosis** _____

A generally benign disease in which functioning endometrial tissue is present in areas outside of the uterine cavity. Severe endometriosis can interfere with conception.

14. **endometritis** _____

Inflammation of the endometrium.

15. **fibroadenoma** _____

Literally, an adenoma (benign tumor) comprised of fibrous tissue. Typically, this describes a benign tumor of the breast.

16. **fibrocystic disease** _____

This is the formation of benign but painful cysts in the breasts.

17. **fibromyoma** _____

Also called a leiomyoma, these are benign tumors that contain both muscular and fibrous components and generally occur in the myometrium layer of the uterus.

18. **gonorrhea** _____

This is a sexually transmitted disease caused by the bacteria Neisseria gonorrhoeae. Symptoms of inflammation, pain, and purulent discharge are more severe in males than females, but it can cause female sterility.

19. **herpes** _____

This refers to any inflammatory skin disease caused by a herpes virus and is characterized by the formation of small clusters of vesicles. Genital herpes (clusters of vesicles which occur on the genitals of both sexes) are transmitted sexually and affect the reproductive system.

Female Reproductive Diseases – Lesson 3

I. **TERMINOLOGY.**
   Enter each term in the space provided. Read the definition and description for each term.

1. **hydatidiform mole** _____

An abnormal pregnancy in which the chorionic villi form a mass of cysts similar in appearance to a cluster of grapes.

2. **infertility** _____

A diminished or absent capacity to produce offspring. This does not refer to the complete inability to produce children, which is called sterility. There are many reasons for infertility and many treatments and procedures available. It is a part of medicine that is advancing and changing rapidly.

3. **leiomyoma** _____

(plural: leiomyomata) A benign tumor derived from the smooth muscle (usually of the uterus). This is also called a fibroid.

4. **mastitis** _____

Inflammation of a mammary gland or the breast.

5. **melasma** _____

Also called the mask of pregnancy. This is a blotchy, brownish color that occurs over the forehead and malar eminence. This brownish pigment is also common around the mammary areola and in a dark line down the abdomen.

6. **nabothian cyst** _____

A small, yellowish mass consisting of dilated endocervical gland and appearing at the external cervical os.

7. **oophoritis** _____

Inflammation of an ovary.

8. **Paget disease** _____

An intraductal carcinoma (cancer) of the breast. Also refers to a neoplasm of the vulva closely associated with Paget disease of the breast, but less likely to become carcinomatous.

9. **placenta previa** _____

This occurs when the placenta implants over or near the internal os of the cervix. If it completely covers the os, it is total previa, and if it only partially covers it, it is a partial previa. It is characterized by sudden, painless vaginal bleeding late in pregnancy.

10. **precocious puberty** _____

The onset of sexual maturation at an earlier age than usual. Incidentally, the lower limit of normal for girls is eight and for boys is nine.

11. **preeclampsia** _____

A complication of pregnancy which is characterized by hypertension, edema, and/or proteinuria.

12. **puerperal infection** _____

Puerperal means pertaining to the period from the end of the third stage of labor until involution of the uterus, which is usually about three to six weeks. A puerperal infection is any infection which afflicts the mother during this time period. Historically, before the discovery of how bacterial infectious processes work, most infant deaths and many maternal deaths associated with childbirth were caused by unclean conditions during labor and delivery. This was called puerperal fever or childbed fever.

13. **salpingitis** _____

Inflammation of a uterine or fallopian tube.

14. **syphilis** _____

A sexually transmitted disease (STD) that passes through three different stages and can be latent for years. It can affect any tissue or organ in the body. Primary symptoms include lesions or rashes and eventually it compromises major body systems.

15. **teratoma** _____

A neoplasm of the ovary which originates from germ cells, or any type of germ cell tumor.

16. **neoplasm** _____

An abnormal growth.

17. **trichomonas** _____

A sexually transmitted disease (STD) that is caused by a parasitic protozoa. Trichomonas vaginalis is found in both the female and male genital tract.

18. **Turner syndrome** _____

A developmental defect in which the ovaries are either absent or represented only by streaks of ovarian tissue in the broad ligaments. Menstruation does not occur.

19. **vaginitis** _____

Inflammation of the vagina that is characterized by pain and purulent discharge.

Male Reproductive System

The same thing that is true of the female reproductive system is true of the male reproductive system: proper function is not vital to the sustenance of a human life, but it is essential to the propagation of the species itself. In other words, if no babies come along, humans will go the way of the dinosaurs! Aside from the obvious differences, there is one major difference in the female and male reproductive systems—the male urethra serves both excretory and reproductive functions as an outlet for both urine and semen.

Male Reproductive Anatomy – Lesson 1

The primary function of the male reproductive system, as stated earlier, is to perpetuate the species. This is done through the creation and transportation of sperm. Most of the structures and organs shown have an important role in this process. The testes (singular: testis) are the male gonads (gamete-producing glands). These are contained in a sac-like structure called the scrotum. Normally there are two testes, each in its own compartment and separated by the longitudinal median septum. Each testis is surrounded by a connective tissue called the tunica albuginea. The testes are further divided into compartments called lobules, which contain the seminiferous tubules where the spermatozoa are produced. The sperm pass from these tubules into the rete testis and then into the efferent ductules to complete the maturation process before leaving the testes.

Male Reproductive Anatomy – Lesson 2

There are two muscles—the dartos (which is part of the scrotal wall) and the cremaster (which is attached to the spermatic cord)—whose function is to respond to temperature fluctuations by regulating the position of the testes within the scrotum. Specifically, cold causes the muscles to contract and the scrotum to elevate and wrinkle; warmth causes the muscles to relax and the scrotum becomes elongated and flaccid.

The epididymis is a very coiled tube that fits snugly over the upper end of each testis. Sperm from the efferent ductules are stored in the epididymis before ejaculation. The total length of the epididymis is 6 to 7 meters. (Yes, that is correct, meters not centimeters).

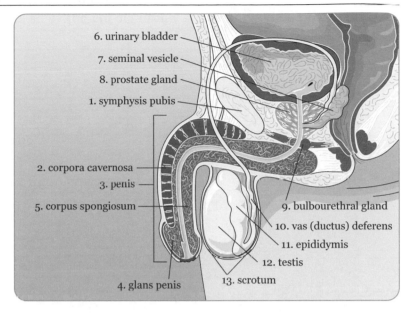

6. urinary bladder
7. seminal vesicle
8. prostate gland
1. symphysis pubis
2. corpora cavernosa
3. penis
5. corpus spongiosum
9. bulbourethral gland
10. vas (ductus) deferens
11. epididymis
12. testis
4. glans penis
13. scrotum

The vas deferens (also called the ductus deferens) is a continuation of the epididymis that ascends to the urethra. It passes out of the scrotum and into the abdominal cavity through an inguinal canal. It is part of the spermatic cord that also includes blood vessels, nerves, and a lining that all function closely with the testis. Once it reaches the abdominal cavity, the vas deferens separates from the rest of the spermatic cord and crosses the ureter to reach the posterior side of the urinary bladder, where it becomes part of the ejaculatory duct. The walls of the lumen of the vas deferens contain muscles and cilia that aid in the movement of the sperm.

The accessory glands, namely the seminal vesicles, prostate gland, and bulbourethral glands, secrete additives to the sperm that strengthen and protect the sperm. These secretions, together with the sperm, are called semen. The seminal vesicles are glands that are found immediately beneath the bladder. They secrete a sticky, alkaline, yellow substance that assists in sperm movement and longevity. It is the union of the seminal vesicles and the vas deferens that make up the ejaculatory ducts. The prostate gland surrounds the urethra at the base of the bladder; this is a singular gland made up of many small glands and muscle fibers enclosed in a dense connective tissue. The prostate secretes a thin, milky, alkaline substance that assists in sperm motility. (The alkaline nature of the seminal fluid protects the sperm from the acidic environment of the female vagina.)

Finally, there are two bulbourethral glands (also called Cowper glands), each approximately the size of a pea, which are located inferior to the prostate. Their ducts open into the urethra where they secrete a mucoid substance before ejaculation that coats the lining of the urethra in order to further protect the sperm.

I. FILL IN THE BLANK.

In the blanks provided below, refer to the image and enter the term corresponding to the following numbers. Use the word(s) in the box to fill in the blanks.

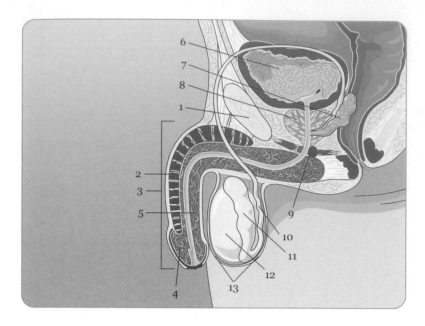

1. _____

2. _____

3. _____

4. _____

5. _____

6. _____

7. _____

8. _____

9. _____

10. _____

11. _____

12. _____

13. _____

prostate gland
corpora cavernosa
epididymis
corpus spongiosum
vas (ductus) deferens
glans penis
seminal vesicle
symphysis pubis
scrotum
bulbourethral gland
penis
testis
urinary bladder

Male Reproductive Anatomy – Lesson 3

The urethra is an approximately 20-cm long S-shaped tube that connects the urinary bladder and ejaculatory ducts to the outside of the body. It is the urethra that differs from the female reproductive system in that it serves both urinary and reproductive systems as a passageway for urine and semen. The urethra continues throughout the length of the penis and enlarges slightly at its end (called the meatus).

The penis is the copulatory organ of the male reproductive system. The penis is anterior to the scrotum, is attached to the pubic arch, and is divided into a tubular shaft and a distal cone-shaped glans. The skin of the penis is hairless, contains no fat cells, and is generally a slightly darker pigment than the rest of the skin. Covering the glans is a loose-fitting, retractable skin called the prepuce or foreskin. The removal of the prepuce is called circumcision. A pair of dorsally positioned masses called the corpora cavernosa penis (singular: corpus cavernosum) is inside the penis, along with a third mass called the corpus spongiosum penis (which is ventral to the other two and surrounds the penile urethra). Finally, there are many dorsal veins along the shaft of the penis.

Ejaculation is the discharge of semen from the penis. In response to stimulation of nerves and vasoconstriction of the veins, there is an increase in blood supply that causes an erection. In this state, the action of the cilia in the lumen of the vas deferens—in combination with contraction of the testes, epididymes, and vasa deferentia—causes semen emission.

On average, approximately 100 million sperm are present in each cubic centimeter of ejaculate. Furthermore, the volume of each ejaculate is 2–4 cubic centimeters. After ejaculation is complete, the blood vessels return to their normal caliber, draining excess blood from the penis and returning it to a flaccid state.

I. MATCHING.
Match the correct term to the definition.

1. ____ urethra

2. ____ penis

3. ____ circumcision

4. ____ ejaculation

5. ____ corpora cavernosa penis

A. The removal of the prepuce or foreskin
B. A pair of dorsally positioned masses inside the penis
C. The tube that connects the urinary bladder and ejaculatory ducts to the outside of the body
D. The discharge of semen from the penis
E. The copulatory organ of the male reproductive system

Male Reproductive Anatomy – Lesson 4

I. TERMINOLOGY.
Enter each term in the space provided. Read the definition and description for each term.

1. **gonads** _____
Gamete-producing glands.

2. **median septum** _____
The separation between the two testes.

3. **tunica albuginea** _____
Connective tissue that surrounds each testis.

4. **seminiferous tubules** _____

The area where the spermatozoa are produced.

5. **rete testis** _____

The network of canals that the sperm run through.

6. **efferent ductules** _____

The area that the rete testis empties into.

7. **dartos** _____

One of the muscles of the scrotal wall that responds to temperature changes and moves the position of the testes within the scrotum.

8. **cremaster** _____

One of the muscles, attached to the spermatic cord, that responds to temperature changes and moves the position of the testes within the scrotum.

9. **spermatic cord** _____

A group of structures that go through the inguinal canal to the testis. The structures include the vas deferens, arteries, veins, lymphatic vessels, and nerves.

10. **semen** _____

The combination of secretions from the seminal vesicles, prostate gland, and bulbourethral glands with sperm.

11. **Cowper gland** _____

Two bulbourethral glands, each approximately the size of a pea, which are located inferior to the prostate.

12. **urethra** _____

A 20-cm long S-shaped tube that connects the urinary bladder and ejaculatory ducts to the outside of the body.

13. **meatus** _____

The end of the urethra.

14. **prepuce** _____

A retractable fold of skin at the tip of the penis, also called foreskin.

15. **circumcision** _____

The removal of the prepuce.

Review: Male Reproductive Anatomy

I. **MULTIPLE CHOICE.**
    Choose the best answer.

1. One of the scrotal wall muscles.
    - ○ dartos
    - ○ urethra
    - ○ rete testis
    - ○ vas deferens

2. Also called bulbourethral glands.
    - ○ tunica albuginea
    - ○ rete testis
    - ○ circumcision
    - ○ Cowper glands

3. The removal of the prepuce.
    - ○ resection
    - ○ epididymis
    - ○ rete testis
    - ○ circumcision

4. Secretions from the glands, in combination with the spermatozoa.
    - ○ sperman
    - ○ seeman
    - ○ semen
    - ○ seman

5. A very coiled tube located at the upper end of each testis that is approximately 6.5 meters in length.
    - ○ epididmis
    - ○ epididymis
    - ○ epididimys
    - ○ epidydimis

6. A continuation of the epididymis that goes up and into the urethra.
    - ○ vas deferens
    - ○ prepuce
    - ○ vasideferens
    - ○ rete testis

7. The foreskin of the penis.

○ glans penis
○ prepuce
○ epididymis
○ dartos

8. The connective tissue that surrounds the testis.

○ tunica albuginea
○ tunica testiculosa
○ tunica spongosa
○ tunica testosterosa

9. The place in the body where the sperm are produced.

○ sperm tubules
○ semen tubules
○ seminiferous tubules
○ epididymis

10. After production, the sperm pass directly into this structure.

○ right testis
○ left testes
○ Cowper glands
○ rete testis

Male Reproductive Diseases

As with any system, there are conditions that negatively affect function in the male reproductive system. Virtually any structure discussed can be afflicted with forms of cancer (adenocarcinoma), become inflamed, or in other ways be impaired. Furthermore, benign neoplasms or tumors can occur in various places throughout the male reproductive system. However, fewer structures make up the male reproductive system compared to systems such as the muscular system or the skeletal system. Keep in mind that the male reproductive system shares structures with the male excretory system and that, consequently, some diseases affect both systems.

The primary symptoms that occur are pain, swelling, tenderness, and/or discoloration of the affected area. Additionally, there are measurements of the prostate gland that are indicative of conditions such as BPH or prostate cancer.

I. TERMINOLOGY.
Enter each term in the space provided. Read the definition and description for each term.

1. **balanitis** _____

Inflammation of the glans penis.

2. **benign prostatic hyperplasia** _____

This term is very often called "benign prostatic hypertrophy" or BPH. It is a condition that often occurs with aging, in which the prostate gland is enlarged two to four times its normal size.

3. **cryptorchidism** _____

Undescended testicle. This is a condition that occurs during fetal development. Failure to correct it before puberty generally causes the affected testicle to atrophy and can lead to an increased chance of malignancy.

4. **epididymitis** _____

Inflammation of the epididymis.

5. **hydrocele** _____

A cystic mass of the spermatic cord, testicle, or both that consists of fluid between the two layers of the tunica vaginalis.

6. **hypospadias** _____

A malformation of the urethra in which the opening is located on the undersurface of the penis instead of the tip. In the condition epispadias, the opening is on the upper surface of the penis.

7. **orchitis** _____

Inflammation of the testicle. This is usually accompanied by epididymitis.

8. **phimosis** _____

The inability of the foreskin to be retracted from the glans penis. The term paraphimosis refers to the inability of the foreskin, once retracted, to be replaced back over the glans.

9. **priapism** _____

Persistent, abnormal penile erection that is not accompanied by either sexual desire or excitation and causes serious pain and tenderness.

10. **prostatitis** _____

Inflammation of the prostate.

11. **spermatocele** _____

A spermatic cyst. This occurs adjacent to the epididymis and usually contains sperm. If it is large, it looks like a "third testis."

12. **torsion** _____

The term torsion means literally a twisting or turning about an axis. Testicular torsion is the most common use of this term, however, and applies specifically to a twisting of the spermatic cord. The condition runs in families, and if it is not corrected the affected area can become gangrenous within hours.

13. **varicocele** _____

A collection of large veins, usually occurring in the left scrotum and described as feeling "like a bag of worms." It is present in the upright position, but empties in the supine position.

Review: Male Reproductive System

I. **MULTIPLE CHOICE.**
   Choose the best answer.

   1. Undescended testicle.
      ○ paraphimosis
      ○ balanitis
      ○ orchitis
      ○ cryptorchidism

   2. The inability of the foreskin to be replaced back over the glans penis.
      ○ varicocele
      ○ priapism
      ○ prostatitis
      ○ paraphimosis

   3. Inflammation of the glans penis.
      ○ benign prostatic hyperplasia
      ○ balanitis
      ○ hypospadias
      ○ hydrocele

   4. A twisting, turning, or rotation about an axis.
      ○ torsion
      ○ torque
      ○ spasm
      ○ priapism

5. A cystic mass of the spermatic cord, testicle, or both.
   - ○ cyst
   - ○ hydrocele
   - ○ fissure
   - ○ varicocele

6. A malformation of the urethra in which the opening is located on the undersurface of the penis.
   - ○ hyperplasia
   - ○ hypourethra
   - ○ hypospadias
   - ○ prostatitis

7. Inflammation of the testicle.
   - ○ testitis
   - ○ inflamitis testicus
   - ○ orchitis
   - ○ prostatitis

8. Persistent abnormal penile erection with no concomitant sexual desire.
   - ○ prostatitis
   - ○ hydrocele
   - ○ penitis
   - ○ priapism

9. A collection of veins which feels like a "bag of worms."
   - ○ varicocele
   - ○ veinocele
   - ○ veinitis
   - ○ varicitis

10. Inflammation of the prostate.
    - ○ prostatogram
    - ○ testitis
    - ○ prostatitis
    - ○ orchitis

11. A condition that occurs with aging, wherein the prostate becomes enlarged.
    ○ hyperprostatitis
    ○ hypospadias
    ○ benign prostatic hyperplasia
    ○ benign prostatic hypotrophy

12. A spermatic cyst, which takes on the appearance of a "third testis."
    ○ varicocele
    ○ spermatocele
    ○ hyperspermitis
    ○ spermatozoa

Answer Key

Anatomy and Disease Basics

Levels of Organization

I. MATCHING.

1. D. made up of several organs which have a common function
2. H. largest structural level
3. B. responsible for all of the movement of the body
4. J. atoms and molecules
5. F. made up of groups of cells and the materials surrounding them
6. I. tissue which is the communication system of the body
7. A. molecules combine together to form this level
8. E. supports posture and function
9. C. protects cavities and organ structures from injury and fluid loss
10. G. tissues combine to form this level

Disease Classification Terms – Lesson 1

II. MATCHING.

1. E. not born with it
2. D. abnormality in development of tissues or organs
3. C. lack or defect
4. B. present at birth
5. A. deteriorating

III. FILL IN THE BLANK.

1. acquired
2. congenital
3. degenerative
4. developmental
5. deficiency

Disease Classification Terms – Lesson 2

II. MATCHING.

1. D. normal structure not working properly; no underlying cause
2. C. of unknown cause OR E. of unknown cause or spontaneous origin
3. A. suggests a hereditary component
4. E. of unknown cause or spontaneous origin OR C. of unknown cause
5. B. transmitted from parent to child

III. FILL IN THE BLANK.

1. essential
2. familial
3. functional
4. idiopathic
5. hereditary

Disease Classification Terms – Lesson 3

II. MATCHING.

1. A. resulting from injury
2. D. caused by dietary intake
3. C. related to a tumor
4. F. caused by infection
5. E. abnormality of a single molecule
6. B. abnormality of a bodily structure

III. FILL IN THE BLANK.

1. nutritional
2. traumatic
3. organic
4. neoplastic
5. infectious
6. molecular

Disease Classification Terms – Lesson 4

II. MATCHING.

1. D. short and severe
2. C. persisting for a long time
3. B. terminal impairment
4. E. having no symptoms
5. A. impairs normal function

III. FILL IN THE BLANK.

1. end-stage
2. disabling
3. acute
4. chronic
5. asymptomatic

Skeletal System

Review: Axial and Appendicular

II. MULTIPLE CHOICE.

1. appendicular
2. appendicular
3. axial
4. axial
5. appendicular
6. appendicular
7. axial
8. appendicular
9. axial
10. axial
11. appendicular
12. axial
13. appendicular
14. appendicular

Review: Function

I. MULTIPLE CHOICE.

1. red blood cells
2. white blood cells
3. carry oxygen from the lungs to the rest of the body
4. help fight infections and aid the immune system
5. reproduce themselves and all other blood cells
6. white blood cells
7. white blood cells
8. mineral
9. rigidity and strength

Bone Formation and Development

I. MATCHING.
1. G. cells that the body has programmed to create bones
2. A. bone-forming cells that secrete a matrix which becomes calcified
3. B. former osteoblasts that are surrounded by bone matrix and have calcified
4. D. the first formation of bone
5. C. large multinucleated cells that reabsorb bone matrix
6. E. bone that has ossified and calcified
7. F. bone formation

II. FILL IN THE BLANK.
1. osteoblasts
2. calcification
3. osteoclasts
4. osteocytes
5. leukocytes
6. bleeding
7. white
8. red
9. 95%
10. appendicular
11. axial
12. hyoid
13. ossification
14. ossification
15. osteoclasts
16. erythropoiesis

Review: Bone Types

II. MULTIPLE CHOICE.
1. Lacunae
2. cancellous
3. compact
4. Canaliculi
5. Osteocytes
6. Marrow
7. immature bone
8. White blood cells

Bone Markings

II. MULTIPLE CHOICE.
1. Bone marking
2. Bone type
3. Bone marking
4. Bone marking
5. Bone type
6. Bone marking
7. Bone type
8. Bone type
9. Bone marking
10. Bone marking
11. Bone type
12. Bone marking
13. Bone type
14. Bone marking
15. Bone marking
16. Bone marking

Main Cranial Bones and Sutures

II. FILL IN THE BLANK.
1. parietal
2. temporal
3. frontal
4. occipital

III. FILL IN THE BLANK.
1. coronal suture
2. sagittal suture
3. lambdoid suture
4. parietal bones
5. frontal bone
6. temporal bone

Review: The Skull

I. FILL IN THE BLANK.

1. coronal suture
2. sphenoid bone
3. nasal bone
4. frontal bone
5. temporal bone
6. nasal concha
7. maxilla
8. parietal bone
9. squamous suture
10. lambdoid suture
11. occipital bone
12. mastoid process
13. styloid process
14. condyloid process
15. coronoid process
16. supraorbital foramen
17. lacrimal bone
18. zygomatic bone
19. vomer
20. mandible

Vertebral Column

II. MATCHING.

1. G. lower back
2. F. between the bones of the spine
3. B. the neck
4. E. connects to the ribs
5. D. join
6. A. triangular shaped
7. C. tailbone

III. FILL IN THE BLANK.

1. lumbar spine
2. articulate
3. cervical spine
4. sacral spine
5. thoracic spine
6. ooocyx
7. intervertebral discs

Review: Axial Skeleton

I. FILL IN THE BLANK.

1. cervical
2. sacral
3. lumbosacral
4. thoracolumbar
5. thoracic
6. intervertebral discs
7. coccyx
8. cervical
9. daggor
10. floating
11. manubrium
12. xiphoid process
13. spinal cord

II. MATCHING.

1. E. 1 bone
2. B. 21 bones
3. A. 26 bones
4. D. 25 bones
5. C. 6 bones
6. F. 7 bones

Shoulder Bones

II. MATCHING.

1. B. collar bone
2. D. where the head of the humerus rests
3. A. upper arm bone
4. E. shoulder blade
5. C. medial end

1. long bone
2. S
3. humerus
4. epicondyle
5. scapula

Arm Bones

II. MATCHING.
1. B. pinky-side bone
2. E. prominence
3. C. point of the elbow
4. D. joint of ulna and radius
5. A. thumb-side bone

III. MULTIPLE CHOICE.
1. ulna
2. radius
3. malleolus
4. tuberosity
5. styloid process

Hand and Wrist Bones

III. MATCHING.
1. C. wrists
2. A. hands
3. B. fingers

Hip Bones and Femur

II. MATCHING.
1. B. thigh bone
2. D. lower part of the "eye mask"
3. C. the head of the femur fits into this
4. E. hip bone
5. A. kneecap

III. MULTIPLE CHOICE.
1. ischium
2. trochanter
3. acetabulum
4. medial and lateral epicondyles
5. femur

Lower Leg and Foot Bones

II. MATCHING.
1. B. feet bones
2. A. ankle bone(s)
3. D. toes
4. E. protects the ankle
5. C. larger lower leg bone

III. MULTIPLE CHOICE.
1. 14
2. fibula
3. tibia
4. epicondyle
5. tibia

Review: Appendicular Skeleton

I. FILL IN THE BLANK.
1. femur
2. patella
3. tibia
4. fibula
5. tarsals
6. metatarsals
7. phalanges
8. clavicle

9. scapula
11. ulna
13. carpals
15. phalanges

10. humerus
12. radius
14. metacarpals

II. FILL IN THE BLANK.

1. sternum
3. metatarsals
5. scapula
7. ribs
9. ulna
11. metacarpals
13. coccyx
15. calcaneal
17. lateral malleolus
19. tibia

2. ischium
4. fibula
6. vertebrae
8. humerus
10. cranium
12. proximal
14. femur
16. humerus
18. ischium
20. transverse arch

III. MATCHING.

1. H. collarbone
3. D. shoulder blade
5. G. fingers and toes
7. A. wrist bones
9. E. kneecap

2. F. strongest bone of the body
4. C. hip bone
6. I. upper arm bone
8. B. ankle bones
10. J. weight-bearing bone of the legs

Joints and Articulations

I. TRUE/FALSE.

1. true
3. false
5. false

2. true
4. true

II. FILL IN THE BLANK.

1. synovial
3. cartilaginous
5. ligaments

2. suture and syndesmosis
4. biaxial

Joint Movement

II. MATCHING.

1. E. unbending
3. C. moving away from midline
5. A. circling

2. B. bending
4. D. adding a part back to the body

III. FILL IN THE BLANK.

1. flexion
3. circumduction
5. adduction

2. extension
4. abduction

V. MATCHING.

1. D. flexing the toe
3. E. around an axis
5. A. lying face down

2. C. pointing the toe
4. B. lying face up

VI. FILL IN THE BLANK.

1. prone
2. rotation
3. plantar flexion
4. dorsiflexion
5. supine

VII. MULTIPLE CHOICE.

1. Movement of the foot that brings the top of the foot closer to the leg.
2. move with ease
3. flexion
4. movement in a circle
5. prone
6. joint
7. fibrous, cartilaginous, synovial
8. synovial joints
9. multiaxial
10. somewhat moveable

Ligaments

II. MATCHING.

1. A. shaped like a cross
2. E. curved or bow-shaped ligament
3. B. support
4. D. like a raven's beak
5. C. indirect

III. FILL IN THE BLANK.

1. coracoid
2. accessory
3. cruciate
4. arcuate
5. collateral

IV. MATCHING.

1. C. sickle-shaped
2. A. the neck
3. F. between bones
4. E. three cornered
5. D. groin area
6. B. lengthwise

V. FILL IN THE BLANK.

1. longitudinal
2. falciform
3. interosseous
4. nuchal
5. triquetral
6. inguinal

Fractures – Lesson 1

II. SPELLING.

1. fragment
2. fracture
3. blow-out
4. butterfly
5. articular

III. MULTIPLE CHOICE.

1. articular
2. comminuted
3. axial
4. apophyseal
5. indirect

Fractures – Lesson 2

II. SPELLING.

1. buttonhole
2. cleavage
3. closed
4. complicated
5. Colles'

III. MATCHING.

1. B. buttonhole
2. E. comminuted
3. A. complete
4. D. Colles'
5. C. chisel

Fractures – Lesson 3

II. SPELLING.

1. condylar
2. dislocation
3. hangman's
4. greenstick
5. axis

III. TRUE/FALSE.

1. false
2. true
3. false
4. true
5. true

Fractures – Lesson 4

II. TRUE/FALSE.

1. true
2. false
3. false
4. false
5. true

III. FILL IN THE BLANK.

1. utero
2. capsule
3. intra-articular
4. density
5. maxilla

Fractures – Lesson 5

II. SPELLING.

1. stress
2. spiral
3. open
4. torus
5. traumatic

III. MULTIPLE CHOICE.

1. torsion
2. subcapital
3. spontaneous
4. transverse
5. tuft

Musculoskeletal Diseases – Lesson 1

II. SPELLING.

1. achondroplasia
2. rheumatoid
3. degenerative
4. inflammation
5. Ewing

III. MULTIPLE CHOICE.

1. cancerous
2. osteoarthritis
3. articular
4. ankylosing
5. joints

Musculoskeletal Diseases – Lesson 2

II. SPELLING.
1. gout
2. mucopolysaccharides
3. alkaline phosphatase
4. Hurler
5. systemic

III. MATCHING.
1. D. gout
2. B. hypophosphatasia
3. E. Legg-Calve-Perthes disease
4. A. Hurler syndrome
5. C. Marfan syndrome

Musculoskeletal Diseases – Lesson 3

II. SPELLING.
1. Osgood-Schlatter
2. osteochondrosis
3. osteochondritis
4. Staphylococcus
5. neoplasm

III. MULTIPLE CHOICE.
1. osteogenesis imperfecta
2. multiple myeloma
3. osteomyelitis
4. osteoid osteoma
5. osteomalacia

Musculoskeletal Diseases – Lesson 4

II. SPELLING.
1. Paget
2. rickets
3. psoriatic
4. Scheuermann
5. arthritis

III. MATCHING.
1. D. kyphosis
2. B. rickets
3. A. Scheuermann disease
4. E. osteoporosis
5. C. scoliosis

Review: Musculoskeletal Diseases

I. MULTIPLE CHOICE.
1. Reiter syndrome
2. scoliosis
3. gout
4. Paget disease
5. achondroplasia

II. MATCHING.
1. B. chondrosarcoma
2. D. hypophosphatasia
3. E. kyphosis
4. H. osteomyelitis
5. A. rickets
6. G. osteoid osteoma
7. F. arthritis
8. C. degenerative joint disease

III. SPELLING.
1. Ewing tumor
2. Legg-Calve-Perthes disease
3. osteogenesis imperfecta
4. kyphosis
5. Reiter syndrome
6. scoliosis
7. rheumatoid
8. psoriatic arthritis

Muscular System

Function and Types

I. MATCHING.

1. D. Allow human skeleton movement
2. F. Maintain a sitting position
3. E. Allow for smooth movement when bending or twisting joints
4. B. When muscles contract and produce heat
5. C. Primary muscles allowing voluntary movement of the body
6. G. Muscles lining the walls of internal organs
7. A. Muscle found only in the heart

Smooth Muscle

I. MULTIPLE CHOICE.

1. resistant to fatigue
2. striations
3. the eye
4. peristalsis
5. greater length than width

Naming Muscles

I. MATCHING.

1. B. Shape
2. C. Location
3. D. Attachment
4. E. Size
5. A. Orientation of fibers
6. G. Relative position
7. F. Function

Anatomical Position

II. MULTIPLE CHOICE.

1. transverse
2. inferior
3. ventral
4. anterior
5. lateral
6. distal
7. proximal
8. medial
9. coronal
10. dorsal
11. ventral
12. posterior

Combining Planes

I. FILL IN THE BLANK.

1. ventrolateral
2. inferoposterior
3. posteroinferior
4. superolateral
5. lateroposterior
6. mediolateral
7. inferomedial
8. superoinferior
9. anteromedial
10. dorsiflexion
11. distocervical
12. anterolateral

Muscles of the Face and Head

I. FILL IN THE BLANK.

1. frontalis
2. temporalis
3. orbicularis oculi
4. buccinator
5. orbicularis oris
6. triangularis
7. corrugator
8. nasalis
9. levator labii superioris
10. greater zygomatic
11. masseter
12. platysma

II. MULTIPLE CHOICE.

1. orbicularis oculi
2. triangularis
3. frontalis
4. platysma
5. buccinator
6. nasalis
7. levator labii superioris
8. orbicularis oris
9. masseter
10. greater zygomatic
11. temporalis
12. corrugator

Muscles of Facial Expression and Mastication

II. SPELLING.

1. mentalis
2. depressor
3. pterygoid
4. labii
5. risorius
6. anguli
7. inferioris

Muscles of the Neck

I. FILL IN THE BLANK.

1. sternocleidomastoid
2. digastric
3. hyoglossus
4. omohyoid
5. sternohyoid

Muscles of the Anterior Torso

I. FILL IN THE BLANK.

1. trapezius
2. deltoid
3. pectoralis major
4. serratus anterior
5. linea alba
6. sternocleidomastoid
7. external oblique
8. umbilicus (belly button) OR umbilicus
9. rectus abdominis

Muscles of the Posterior Torso

I. FILL IN THE BLANK.

1. trapezius
2. deltoid
3. infraspinatus
4. teres minor
5. teres major
6. latissimus dorsi
7. gluteus medius
8. supraspinatus
9. rhomboideus (major)
10. erector spinae group
11. lumbar aponeurosis

Muscles of the Arm

I. FILL IN THE BLANK.

1. coracobrachialis
2. brachialis
3. hypothenar muscles
4. palmar aponeurosis
5. abductor pollicis brevis
6. flexor retinaculum
7. palmaris longus
8. flexor carpi radialis
9. brachioradialis
10. biceps brachii
11. triceps
12. flexor carpi ulnaris
13. flexor digitorum superficialis

Deep Muscles of the Arm

I. TRUE/FALSE.

1. false
2. true
3. true
4. false

Actions of Arm Muscles

II. MULTIPLE CHOICE.

1. supinate
2. pollex
3. anconeus
4. extensor digiti minimi
5. thenar
6. brevis
7. coracobrachialis
8. retinaculum
9. biceps
10. pronator teres
11. extensor digitorum communis
12. palmaris longus
13. triceps
14. flexor digitorum profundus

Muscles of the Leg

I. FILL IN THE BLANK

1. adductor magnus
2. semitendinosus
3. semimembranosus
4. soleus
5. calcaneal (Achilles) tendon OR calcaneal tendon
6. gluteus maximus
7. greater trochanter
8. iliotibial tract
9. biceps femoris
10. peroneus longus
11. peroneus brevis

II. FILL IN THE BLANK.

1. tensor fasciae latae
2. sartorius
3. rectus femoris
4. vastus lateralis
5. iliopsoas
6. pectineus
7. adductor longus
8. gracilis
9. vastus medialis
10. gastrocnemius
11. soleus
12. extensor retinaculum

Muscles of the Lower Leg

I. FILL IN THE BLANK.
1. peroneus longus
2. peroneus brevis
3. lateral malleolus
4. extensor digitorum longus
5. anterior tibialis
6. tibia
7. gastrocnemius
8. soleus
9. extensor hallucis longus
10. medial malleolus

Review: Muscle Anatomy

I. FILL IN THE BLANK.
1. face
2. arm
3. leg
4. face
5. neck
6. face
7. arm
8. back
9. face
10. face
11. arm
12. arm
13. back OR torso
14. neck OR face
15. neck
16. arm
17. arm
18. face
19. back
20. leg
21. leg
22. face
23. leg
24. arm
25. face
26. face
27. leg
28. face
29. leg
30. torso
31. neck
32. arm
33. leg
34. leg
35. face
36. leg
37. leg
38. back
39. face
40. torso
41. arm
42. back
43. leg

II. MULTIPLE CHOICE.
1. pronator teres
2. biceps
3. mentalis
4. gluteus maximus
5. extensor digiti minimi
6. extensor hallucis longus
7. lumbar aponeurosis
8. rhomboideus
9. deltoid
10. lateral and medial pterygoid
11. lateral malleolus
12. levator labii superioris
13. triceps
14. external oblique
15. orbicularis oris
16. Achilles tendon
17. greater trochanter
18. superolateral
19. semimembranosus
20. proprioception
21. flexor carpi radialis
22. gracilis
23. biceps femoris
24. gluteus medius
25. brevis
26. musculoskeletal system
27. posteroanterior

Muscular Diseases

I. MULTIPLE CHOICE.

1. orthopedists
3. clonic activity

2. a seizure
4. neurological, but manifests in the musculoskeletal system

Digestive System

Mouth and Associated Organs

I. FILL IN THE BLANK.

1. labia
3. oral cavity proper
5. red margin
7. labial frenulum

2. vestibule
4. stratified squamous epithelium
6. vermilion border

Palate

II. FILL IN THE BLANK.

1. gingivae (gums)
3. uvula
5. inferior labial frenulum
7. superior labia (upper lip)
9. posterior wall oropharynx
11. vestibule

2. hard palate
4. gingivae (gums)
6. superior labial frenulum
8. soft palate
10. tongue
12. inferior labia (lower lip)

III. MULTIPLE CHOICE.

1. viscera
3. oral cavity
5. gut

2. lumen
4. buccal
6. abdomen

Anatomy of the Tongue

II. FILL IN THE BLANK.

1. lingual tonsils
3. fungiform papillae OR fungiform papillae (large bumps)
5. lingual tonsils
7. filiform papillae OR filiform papillae (small bumps)

2. circumvallate papillae
4. epiglottis

6. sulcus terminalis

III. MULTIPLE CHOICE.

1. papillae
3. lingual frenulum

2. lingual

Salivary Glands

I. MULTIPLE CHOICE.
1. water, ions, mucus, and enzymes
2. growth of good bacteria
3. all of the above
4. when we eat or anticipate eating
5. on the tongue, palate, lips, and cheeks

Teeth

II. FILL IN THE BLANK.
1. crown
2. neck
3. root canal
4. root
5. enamel
6. dentin
7. dentin tubules
8. pulp cavity
9. gingiva
10. cementum
11. bone

Alimentary Canal

II. FILL IN THE BLANK.
1. tunica mucosa
2. tunica submucosa
3. tunica muscularis
4. tunica serosa

Structures of the Alimentary Canal

I. MULTIPLE CHOICE.
1. parietal peritoneum
2. gastroenterology
3. serosa
4. absorption
5. omentum
6. secretion
7. serosa
8. alimentary canal
9. muscularis
10. retroperitoneal
11. dorsal mesentery
12. 30 feet
13. submucosa
14. distention
15. collagen
16. peristalsis
17. secretory
18. greater omentum
19. support

Review: Upper Digestive Structures

I. SPELLING.
1. papillae
2. gastroenterology
3. distention
4. lingual
5. peritoneum
6. mucosa
7. mesentery
8. omentum
9. lumen
10. peristalsis

II. MATCHING.
1. G. tunica adventitia
2. B. omentum
3. D. lumen
4. J. retroperitoneal
5. A. oral cavity
6. F. abdomen
7. E. greater omentum
8. C. gut
9. I. lingual
10. H. buccal

III. MULTIPLE CHOICE.

1. gastroenterology
2. parietal peritoneum
3. papillae
4. viscera
5. absorption
6. lingual frenulum
7. collagen
8. peristalsis
9. 30 feet
10. support

Major Structures of the Digestive System

II. FILL IN THE BLANK.

1. pharynx
2. liver
3. gallbladder
4. duodenum
5. ascending colon
6. cecum
7. appendix
8. rectum
9. parotid (salivary) gland
10. esophagus
11. stomach
12. pancreas
13. transverse colon
14. descending colon
15. sigmoid colon
16. small intestine

Mouth and Esophagus

I. MATCHING.

1. E. passageway for the respiratory and digestive system
2. A. small, fleshy mass hanging from the soft palate
3. C. extends from the soft palate in the mouth to the level of the hyoid bone
4. B. lid-like structure that hangs over the entrance to the larynx
5. D. part of the alimentary canal that connects the pharynx to the stomach

Stomach

I. TRUE/FALSE.

1. false
2. false
3. true
4. false
5. true

Small Intestine and Large Intestine

I. TRUE/FALSE.

1. false
2. true
3. true

II. FILL IN THE BLANK.

1. sigmoid colon
2. cecum
3. hepatic flexure
4. splenic flexure
5. anal canal
6. rectum

Large Organs of the Digestive System

I. FILL IN THE BLANK.

1. pancreas
2. teniae coli
3. liver
4. gallbladder

1. anal canal
2. rectum
3. sigmoid colon
4. descending colon
5. transverse colon
6. ascending colon
7. cecum
8. appendix
9. sacculations or haustra

Review: Digestive Structures

II. MULTIPLE CHOICE.

1. splenic flexure
2. sacculations
3. bolus
4. fundus
5. uvula
6. duodenum
7. ileocecal valve
8. splenic flexure
9. rectum
10. appendix
11. epiglottis
12. stomach
13. esophagus
14. cecum

III. FILL IN THE BLANK.

1. pharynx
2. liver
3. gallbladder
4. duodenum
5. ascending colon
6. cecum
7. appendix
8. rectum
9. parotid (salivary) gland
10. esophagus
11. stomach
12. pancreas
13. transverse colon
14. descending colon
15. sigmoid colon
16. small intestine

Symptoms of Gastrointestinal Illness

II. MULTIPLE CHOICE.

1. tenesmus
2. afebrile
3. regurgitation
4. haustra
5. sphincter
6. constipation
7. heartburn
8. bolus
9. borborygmi
10. pallor
11. weakness
12. flatulence
13. anorexia
14. hematochezia
15. febrile
16. odynophagia
17. melena
18. hematemesis
19. nausea
20. vomiting
21. obstipation
22. dysphagia

Gastrointestinal Disorders – Lesson 1

II. SPELLING.

1. cholecystitis
2. vermiform
3. cheiloschisis
4. anorexia nervosa OR nervosa
5. appendicitis

III. MULTIPLE CHOICE.

1. achalasia
2. bezoar
3. botulism
4. atresia
5. cholelithiasis

Gastrointestinal Disorders – Lesson 2

II. MULTIPLE CHOICE.
1. diverticula
2. caries
3. diverticulosis
4. Zenker
5. cirrhosis

III. MATCHING.
1. A. colitis
2. D. dehydration
3. C. diarrhea
4. B. diverticulum
5. E. diverticulitis

Gastrointestinal Disorders – Lesson 3

II. MULTIPLE CHOICE.
1. fecalith
2. dysentery
3. amebiasis
4. esophagitis
5. dyspepsia

III. TRUE/FALSE.
1. false
2. true
3. true
4. false
5. false

Gastrointestinal Disorders – Lesson 4

II. SPELLING.
1. gastritis
2. halitosis
3. hepatitis
4. gastroenteritis
5. gastroesophageal reflux disease OR reflux

III. MATCHING.
1. C. hernia
2. A. paraesophageal hiatal
3. B. hiatal
4. E. sliding hiatal
5. D. abdominal

Gastrointestinal Disorders – Lesson 5

II. MULTIPLE CHOICE.
1. umbilical hernia
2. intussusception
3. Hirschsprung disease
4. Crohn disease
5. adynamic ileus

III. TRUE/FALSE.
1. false
2. true
3. true
4. false
5. false

Gastrointestinal Disorders – Lesson 6

II. MULTIPLE CHOICE.
1. pancreatitis
2. Giardia
3. malabsorption
4. leukoplakia
5. jaundice

1. B. giardiasis   2. C. irritable bowel syndrome
3. A. mumps   4. E. parasite
5. D. obstruction

Gastrointestinal Disorders – Lesson 7

II. SPELLING.

1. pruritus ani OR pruritus
2. pharyngitis
3. Barrett esophagus
4. peptic
5. ulcer

III. MULTIPLE CHOICE.

1. Schatzki
2. volvulus
3. peritoneum
4. sessile
5. polyp

Bacteria Affecting the Digestive System

II. SPELLING.

1. Clostridium perfringens
2. Shigella dysenteriae
3. Escherichia coli
4. Salmonella
5. Clostridium difficile
6. Staphylococcus aureus
7. Campylobacter
8. Helicobacter pylori
9. Shigella boydii
10. Enterobacter

Respiratory System

Respiration

II. FILL IN THE BLANK.

1. sinuses
2. oral cavity
3. epiglottis
4. thyroid cartilage
5. vocal folds
6. esophagus
7. trachea
8. lungs
9. heart
10. diaphragm

Gross Respiratory Anatomy

I. FILL IN THE BLANK.

1. nasal cavity
2. external naris
3. larynx
4. trachea
5. right pulmonary bronchus
6. hard palate
7. soft palate
8. pharynx
9. lungs
10. left pulmonary bronchus

II. FILL IN THE BLANK.

1. lower
2. upper
3. upper
4. lower
5. upper
6. upper
7. lower
8. lower
9. upper
10. upper

Nasal Cavity

II. TRUE/FALSE.

1. true
2. false
3. true

Sinus Cavities

I. FILL IN THE BLANK.

1. frontal sinuses
2. ethmoid sinus cells
3. maxillary sinuses
4. turbinates

Pharynx

I. FILL IN THE BLANK.

1. laryngopharynx
2. nasopharynx
3. pharynx
4. oropharynx

Larynx and Trachea

II. FILL IN THE BLANK.

1. hyoid bone
2. thyrohyoid membrane
3. thyroid cartilage
4. trachea

III. FILL IN THE BLANK.

1. hyoid bone
2. epiglottis
3. thyroid cartilage
4. esophagus
5. trachea

Bronchi

II. FILL IN THE BLANK.

1. trachea
2. bronchial tubes
3. secondary bronchus
4. tertiary bronchus

Lungs

I. FILL IN THE BLANK.

1. upper lobe
2. superior vena cava
3. aorta
4. middle lobe
5. lower lobe

Pulmonology

II. MULTIPLE CHOICE.
1. pulmonology
2. inspiration
3. diffusion
4. ventilation
5. incentive spirometry
6. diaphragm
7. expiration

Respiratory Symptoms

II. FILL IN THE BLANK.
1. symptom
2. part
3. symptom
4. symptom
5. part
6. symptom
7. symptom
8. part
9. part
10. symptom
11. part
12. symptom
13. part
14. part

Assessing Respiratory Symptoms

I. FILL IN THE BLANK.
1. auscultation
2. percussion
3. hypoxia OR hypoxemia
4. anoxia
5. hypercapnia
6. thoracentesis
7. bronchoscopy

II. MULTIPLE CHOICE.
1. cough
2. auscultation
3. hemoptysis
4. hypoxemia
5. tachypnea
6. hypercapnia
7. stridor
8. percussion
9. purulent
10. congestion
11. cyanosis
12. dyspnea
13. bronchoscopy
14. thoracentesis

Common Respiratory Problems – Lesson 1

II. SPELLING.
1. asphyxia
2. apnea
3. bronchiectasis
4. expectoration
5. paroxysmal

III. MULTIPLE CHOICE.
1. abscess
2. adult respiratory distress syndrome
3. atelectasis
4. asthma
5. fetid

Common Respiratory Problems – Lesson 2

II. SPELLING.

1. epiglottitis
2. bronchiolitis
3. bronchopneumonitis
4. coccidioidomycosis
5. bronchitis

III. MATCHING.

1. C. bronchoalveolitis
2. A. empyema
3. E. chronic obstructive airway disease
4. B. bronchopneumonia
5. D. emphysema

Common Respiratory Problems – Lesson 3

II. MULTIPLE CHOICE.

1. hemothorax
2. hyaline membrane disease
3. infiltrate
4. papilloma
5. epistaxis

III. MULTIPLE CHOICE.

1. hyperventilation
2. interstitial
3. laryngitis
4. pertussis
5. pleural

Common Respiratory Problems – Lesson 4

II. SPELLING.

1. asbestosis
2. serous
3. sanguineous
4. berylliosis
5. silicosis

III. MULTIPLE CHOICE.

1. pneumoconiosis
2. serosanguineous
3. pleurisy
4. anthracosis
5. serous

Common Respiratory Problems – Lesson 5

II. MULTIPLE CHOICE.

1. Pseudomonas aeruginosa
2. consolidation
3. Pneumococcus pneumoniae
4. Klebsiella pneumoniae
5. Legionnaires' disease

III. MATCHING.

1. A. pneumonitis
2. D. Acinetobacter
3. B. Hemophilus influenzae
4. E. Legionella pneumophila
5. C. Mycoplasma pneumoniae

Common Respiratory Problems – Lesson 6

II. SPELLING.

1. rhinorrhea
2. Boeck sarcoid
3. Streptococcus pneumoniae
4. tonsillitis
5. sarcoidosis

III. MULTIPLE CHOICE.

1. Staphylococcus aureus
2. pneumothorax
3. rhinitis
4. sinusitis
5. granulomatous

Common Respiratory Problems – Lesson 7

II. SPELLING.

1. Mycobacterium
2. Wegener's granulomatosis
3. tracheitis
4. tuberculosis
5. granulomatosis

III. MULTIPLE CHOICE.

1. tracheitis
2. Mycobacterium tuberculosis
3. Wegener's granulomatosis
4. upper respiratory infection
5. tuberculosis

Reproductive System

Female Reproductive System

I. FILL IN THE BLANK.

1. fallopian tube
2. fimbria
3. follicle
4. vagina
5. cervix
6. endometrium
7. myometrium
8. ovary
9. perimetrium

II. FILL IN THE BLANK.

1. uterus
2. urinary bladder
3. symphysis pubis
4. clitoris
5. labium minus
6. labium majus
7. rectum

Internal Female Organs

II. MULTIPLE CHOICE.

1. myometrium
2. the secretory stage when the glands become large and coiled
3. 1
4. fornix

External Female Organs

I. TRUE/FALSE.

1. false
2. true
3. true
4. true
5. false

II. FILL IN THE BLANK.
   1. fatty tissue
   3. areola
   5. lobules

   2. milk ducts
   4. nipple

Review: Female Reproduction

I. MULTIPLE CHOICE.
   1. graafian follicle
   3. external genitalia
   5. infundibulum
   7. ampulla
   9. fundus
   11. mesentery
   13. estrogen
   15. mesovarium
   17. corpus luteum
   19. menstruation
   21. lactation
   23. cortex
   25. oviducts
   27. secretory phase

   2. mons pubis
   4. prepuce
   6. areola
   8. stroma
   10. vulva
   12. Bartholin gland
   14. sebaceous
   16. medulla
   18. perineum
   20. menses
   22. mammary glands
   24. fornix
   26. symphysis pubis
   28. gametes or ova

Assessing Female Reproductive System

I. FILL IN THE BLANK.
   1. Pap smear
   3. menarche
   5. hysterosalpingogram

   2. luteal phase
   4. bimanual examination
   6. estradiol

Pregnancy

I. MATCHING.
   1. E. the hormone that indicates pregnancy in the blood or urine
   3. B. pregnancy outcome
   5. C. a test indicating defects and chromosomal abnormalities

   2. A. pregnant woman
   4. D. indicates voluntary or spontaneous loss

Childbirth

I. MULTIPLE CHOICE.
   1. breech
   3. effacement
   5. episiotomy
   7. Apgar
   9. postpartum

   2. lochia
   4. amniotomy
   6. station
   8. placenta
   10. centimeters

Male Reproductive Anatomy – Lesson 2

I. FILL IN THE BLANK.

1. symphysis pubis
2. corpora cavernosa
3. penis
4. glans penis
5. corpus spongiosum
6. urinary bladder
7. seminal vesicle
8. prostate gland
9. bulbourethral gland
10. vas (ductus) deferens
11. epididymis
12. testis
13. scrotum

Male Reproductive Anatomy – Lesson 3

I. MATCHING.

1. C. The tube that connects the urinary bladder and ejaculatory ducts to the outside of the body
2. E. The copulatory organ of the male reproductive system
3. A. The removal of the prepuce or foreskin
4. D. The discharge of semen from the penis
5. B. A pair of dorsally positioned masses inside the penis

Review: Male Reproductive Anatomy

I. MULTIPLE CHOICE.

1. dartos OR cremaster
2. Cowper glands
3. circumcision
4. semen
5. epididymis
6. vas deferens
7. prepuce
8. tunica albuginea
9. seminiferous tubules
10. rete testis

Review: Male Reproductive System

I. MULTIPLE CHOICE.

1. cryptorchidism
2. paraphimosis
3. balanitis
4. torsion
5. hydrocele
6. hypospadias
7. orchitis
8. priapism
9. varicocele
10. prostatitis
11. benign prostatic hyperplasia
12. spermatocele